POULTRY FEATHERS AND SKIN

The Poultry Integument in Health and Welfare

Poultry Science Symposium Series

Executive Editor (Volumes 1–18): B.M. Freeman

1 Physiology of the Domestic Fowl*
2 Protein Utilization by Poultry*
3 Environmental Control in Poultry Production*
4 Egg Quality – a Study of the Hen's Egg*
5 The Fertility and Hatchability of the Hen's Egg*
6 i. Factors Affecting Egg Grading*
ii. Aspects of Poultry Behaviour*
7 Poultry Disease and World Economy
8 Egg Formation and Production
9 Energy Requirements of Poultry*
10 Economic Factors Affecting Egg Production*
11 Digestion in the Fowl*
12 Growth and Poultry Meat Production*
13 Avian Coccidiosis*
14 Food Intake Regulation in Poultry*
15 Meat Quality in Poultry and Game Birds
16 Avian Immunology
17 Reproductive Biology of Poultry
18 Poultry Genetics and Breeding
19 Nutrient Requirements of Poultry and Nutritional Research*
20 Egg Quality – Current Problems and Recent Advances*
21 Recent Advances in Turkey Science
22 Avian Incubation
23 Bone Biology and Skeletal Disorders
24 Poultry Immunology*
25 Poultry Meat Science
26 Poultry Feedstuffs
27 Welfare of the Laying Hen
28 Avian Gut Function in Health and Disease
29 Biology of Breeding Poultry
30 Alternative Systems for Poultry: Health, Welfare and Productivity
31 Sustainable Poultry Production in Europe
32 Poultry Feathers and Skin: The Poultry Integument in Health and Welfare

*Out of print
Volumes 1–24 were not published by CAB International. Those still in print may be ordered from:

Carfax Publishing Company
PO Box 25, Abingdon, Oxfordshire OX14 3UE, UK

Poultry Feathers and Skin

The Poultry Integument in Health and Welfare

Poultry Science Symposium Series
Volume Thirty Two

Edited by

Oluyinka A. Olukosi
University of Georgia, USA

Victor E. Olori
Aviagen Limited, UK

Ariane Helmbrecht
Evonik Nutrition and Care, GmbH

Sarah Lambton
University of Bristol, UK

and

Nick A. French
Aviagen Limited, UK

CABI

CABI is a trading name of CAB International

CABI
Nosworthy Way
Wallingford
Oxfordshire OX10 8DE
UK
Tel: +44 (0)1491 832111
Fax: +44 (0)1491 833508
E-mail: info@cabi.org
Website: www.cabi.org

CABI
745 Atlantic Avenue
8th Floor
Boston, MA 02111
USA
T: +1 (617) 682 9015
E-mail: cabi-nao@cabi.org

A catalogue record for this book is available from the British Library, London, UK.

Library of Congress Cataloging-in-Publication Data

Names: Olukosi, Oluyinka A., editor.
Title: Poultry feathers and skin : the poultry integument in health and welfare / editors, Oluyinka A. Olukosi, University of Georgia, USA, Victor E. Olori, Aviagen Limited, UK, Ariane Helmbrecht, Evonik Nutrition and Care, GmbH, Sarah Lambton, University of Bristol, UK, Nick A. French, Aviagen Limited, UK.
Description: Wallingford, Oxfordshire, UK : CABI, [2019] | Series: Poultry science symposium series ; volume 32 | Includes bibliographical references and index.
Identifiers: LCCN 2018049623 (print) | LCCN 2018050038 (ebook) | ISBN 9781786395139 (ePDF) | ISBN 9781786395122 (ePub) | ISBN 9781786395121 (epub) ISBN 9781786395115 (hbk : alk. paper)
Subjects: LCSH: Poultry--Physiology. | Feathers--Physiology. | Skin--Physiology.
Classification: LCC SF768.2.P6 (ebook) | LCC SF768.2.P6 P68 2019 (print) | DDC 636.5--dc23

LC record available at https://lccn.loc.gov/2018049623

ISBN-13: 978 1 78639 511 5 (hardback)
978 1 78639 513 9 (ePDF)
978 1 78639 512 2 (ePub)

Commissioning editor: Alex Lainsbury
Editorial assistant: Emma McCann
Production editor: Tim Kapp and Ali Thompson

Typeset by AMA DataSet, Preston, UK.
Printed and bound in the UK by Bell & Bain Ltd, Glasgow.

CONTENTS

CONTRIBUTORS

Sunday A. Adedokun, *Department of Animal and Food Science, University of Kentucky, Lexington, KY 40546, USA. E-mail: tayo.adedokun@uky.edu*

Piter Bijma, *Animal Breeding and Genomics, Wageningen University & Research, P.O. Box 338, 6700 AH Wageningen, Netherlands. E-mail: piter.bijma@wur.nl*

Avigdor Cahaner, *The Hebrew University, Faculty of Agriculture, Rehovot 76100, Israel. E-mail: avigdor.cahaner@mail.huji.ac.il*

Esther D. Ellen, *Animal Breeding and Genomics, Wageningen University & Research, P.O. Box 338, 6700 AH, Wageningen, the Netherlands. E-mail: esther.ellen@wur.nl*

Denis Headon, *Roslin Institute and Royal (Dick) School of Veterinary Studies, University of Edinburgh, Easter Bush, EH25 9RG, UK. E-mail: denis.headon@roslin.ed.ac.uk*

Paul M. Hocking, *formerly of the Roslin Institute and Royal (Dick) School of Veterinary Studies, University of Edinburgh, Easter Bush, EH25 9RG, UK.*

Dagmar N.R.G. Kapell, *Aviagen Ltd, Newbridge, Midlothian EH28 8SZ, UK. E-mail: dkapell@aviagen.com*

Theagarten Lingham-Soliar, *Nelson Mandela Metropolitan University, Port Elizabeth, South Africa. E-mail: theagarjen.soliar@nmmu.ac.za*

Stephen Lister, *Crowshall Veterinary Services, 1 Crows Hall Lane, Attleborough, NR17 1AD, UK. E-mail: salister@crowshall.co.uk*

Paul F. McMullin, *Poultry Health Services, Marsh Lane, Hemingford Grey, Huntingdon, Cambridgeshire, PE28 9EN. Email: paulmcmullin@poultryhealthinternational.com*

Christine J. Nicol, *The Royal Veterinary College, University of London, Hawkshead Lane, North Mymms, Hatfield, Hertfordshire, AL9 7TA, UK. E-mail: cnicol@rvc.ac.uk*

Opeyemi C. Olojede, *Department of Animal and Food Sciences, University of Kentucky, Lexington, KY 40546, USA. E-mail: ocol223@uky.edu*

Victor E. Olori, *Aviagen Ltd, Newbridge, Midlothian, EH28 8SZ, UK. E-mail: veolori@aviagen.com*

Rick A. van Emous, *Wageningen Livestock Research, P.O. Box 338, 6700 AH Wageningen, Netherlands. E-mail: rick.vanemous@wur.nl*

Marinus M. van Krimpen, *Wageningen Livestock Research, P.O. Box 338, 6700 AH Wageningen, Netherlands. E-mail: marinus.vankrimpen@wur.nl*

Thea van Niekerk, *Wageningen Livestock Research, P.O. Box 338, 6700 AH Wageningen, Netherlands. E-mail: thea.vanniekerk@wur.nl*
Otto A. van Tuijl, *Jannelandseweg 17, 4661 GC Halsteren, Netherlands. E-mail: otto.van.tuijl@planet.nl*
Teun Veldkamp, *Wageningen Livestock Research, P.O. Box 338, 6700 AH Wageningen; De Elst 1, 6708 WD Wageningen, Netherlands. E-mail: teun.veldkamp@wur.nl*

Foreword

The integument is essential for the health and welfare of all poultry species and includes one of the most complex structures in all vertebrates and unique to birds: the feather. The feather has many functions in birds, including flight, thermal insulation, protection and courtship display. In poultry, the most important functions of feathers are to protect the skin from physical damage and to help keep the bird warm. Poor feather cover results in increased incidence of skin damage, contact dermatitis, pecking damage, increased heat loss and, in breeders, a reluctance to mate, all leading to poor bird welfare and reduced profitability for the poultry producer.

While good skin and feather quality is important for the poultry industry, research on the factors that affect skin and feather development is limited and often an incidental part of studies on other issues. The objective of the symposium 'Poultry Feathers and Skin: The Poultry Integument in Health and Welfare' held in Cambridge, UK on 3–5 July 2017 was to bring together poultry experts to review the available information and perhaps to identify where further research was required. This book contains the resulting reviews covering the available scientific literature on the poultry integument and it is an essential reference for poultry science researchers, students and poultry practitioners

The book starts by discussing the development, structure and function of skin and feathers in birds (Part I). Part II covers various factors affecting feather pecking, an important welfare issue for poultry species. This part also discusses contact and foot pad dermatitis and diseases of the skin. The genetics of feather form and colour and the effects of selecting against contact dermatitis are covered in Part III. The concluding Part IV discusses the importance of nutrition for feather development, and good gut health for maintaining litter quality and reducing dermatitis. The effect of poultry management practice on feather loss in broiler breeders as well as the business opportunities for using poultry skin and feathers are also covered in this section. One of the clear messages to come from these papers was that good poultry management, nutrition and disease control were an essential part of maintaining feathers and skin integrity and to minimize health and welfare issues.

This book is the 32nd volume of the Poultry Science Symposium Series produced by the UK Branch of the World's Poultry Science Association. The editors would like to thank all the authors for their contribution to the symposium, the symposium organizing committee for all their hard work in ensuring the symposium was a success, and the sponsors for their generous support.

PREFACE

The feathers – a unique and complex structure of the poultry integument – fulfil diverse tasks like flight, thermal insulation, protection and courtship display. However, in commercial poultry, feathers are additionally of economic interest. In order to discuss the commercial relevance of good and healthy skin and feathers, the 32nd Poultry Science Symposium organized by the UK Branch of the World's Poultry Science Association attended to the objective 'Poultry Feathers and Skin: The Poultry Integument in Health and Welfare'. This book collects the discussed topics starting from the structure and function of skin and feathers, the embryonic development of the integument, factors affecting feather pecking, contact and foot pad dermatitis, diseases of the skin, genetics of feather form and colour as well as the effects of selecting against contact dermatitis, but also the importance of good nutrition for feather development, gut health in regard to litter quality and dermatitis as well as the effect of management on feather loss and business opportunities for using poultry skin and feather.

Dedication

Dr Paul Hocking 1948–2018

Sadly, Paul Hocking, one of the contributors to the symposium, passed away on 25 July 2018 after a brave fight against cancer. Paul's chapter in this book was one of the last of his many distinguished contributions to poultry science.

Paul's career started as a cattle geneticist, obtaining a PhD at Reading University. It was while he was at the Animal Research Centre in Ottawa that he first started to get interested in poultry. In 1983, Paul joined the Poultry Research Centre in Edinburgh and started working on poultry reproduction, trying to understand the broiler breeder paradox. Throughout Paul's career at the Poultry Research Centre, later to become The Roslin Institute and eventually part of the University of Edinburgh, he undertook research in a wide range of poultry science subjects, including factors affecting contact dermatitis. Paul authored or co-authored over 200 papers and was editor of two of the preceding volumes in this symposium series: *Biology of Breeding Poultry* (2009) and *Alternative Systems for Poultry: Health, Welfare and Productivity* (2012).

Paul made a significant contribution to the UK Branch of the World Poultry Science Association (WPSA), serving as President, and to the European Federation of WPSA, where he was Vice-President of Working Group 3 (Genetics). He had a long involvement with *British Poultry Science* and became its Joint Editor. In 2016, Paul's contribution to poultry science was recognized when he was elected to the International Poultry Hall of Fame.

Paul will be much missed, both as a poultry scientist and a friend, by all those who knew him.

Acknowledgements

The support for this symposium is gratefully acknowledged from the following organizations: ABN, Aviagen Group, Evonik Industries, Hendrix Genetics, Premier Nutrition, World's Poultry Science Association (WPSA) (UK branch), Zinpro and Zoetis.

PART I

About the Feather and Its Development

CHAPTER 1
The Feather, a Triumph of Natural Engineering and Multifunctionality

Theagarten Lingham-Soliar*
Nelson Mandela University, South Campus, Port Elizabeth, South Africa

ABSTRACT

Structures in nature have evolved over millions of years and, unlike in engineering, are multifunctional. For example, an airplane wing may perform only a single function: lift. This is unlike the bird wing which, besides also producing power, has an ability to detect local updraught information along the entire surface of the wing such as changes in the distribution of pressure that are vital to soaring and energy saving. This chapter demonstrates how multifunctionality of the feather has enabled vital aspects of bird life. Three of these, involving flight, protection and temperature control, are discussed.

The feather is a structure central to bird flight and the rachis is the central structure of the feather. Syncytial barbule fibres in the rachis are long continuous strands with intermittent hooked nodes, which contribute with the matrix to form the most effective bonding mechanisms known in nature. The unique microstructure of feathers that has enabled flight has also contributed to a tough outer integument that protects the bird against predators and the environment. Feathers are organized into tracts or pterylae with spaces, the apteria. This system of feather arrangement enables a dense layering of the feathers for mechanical protection without impeding movement. The apteria also help to reduce the total weight of the feathering, which is important for flight.

The precise design of the barbule with nodes and hooks is fundamental to the process of thermoregulation in down feathers. The embryonic down feathers of chicks form individual 'clumps' of more or less circular masses that have a tree-like, highly organized self-similar structure, which is crucial to its thermal properties. Each tree-like assemblage comprises a barb and branching barbules, described as primary and secondary structures, attached to the skin by a quill. The whole structure creates a 'fluffiness' that helps to trap the warm air.

*theagarten.soliar@nmmu.ac.za

INTRODUCTION

When vertebrates moved on to land hundreds of millions of years ago, one of the major changes involved a fundamental development of the skin with – for the first time – a distinctive epidermis and the development of a complete body covering of scales. The epidermis was capable of providing mechanical protection, preventing desiccation and providing ultraviolet protection, which together with the dermis provided a double layer of protection. The momentous development was in the composition of the scales of an entirely new material: β-keratin, which is extremely tough and stable and, critically, extremely lightweight. The properties of β-keratin would be applied to the development of the feather and it is probably safe to say that bird flight would not have evolved were it not for this material (Lingham-Soliar, 2014b). Most aspects of bird life are inextricably linked to feather structure and evolution. This chapter looks at the role the feather has played in three vital and fundamental aspects of bird life: flight, protection and thermoregulation.

FEATHERS AND FLIGHT

The arrangement of wing feathers (remiges) and tail feathers (rectrices) is shown for a bird of prey (Fig. 1.1).

The longest wing feathers are the primaries, which extend from the carpal ('wrist') joint towards the wing tip (Fig. 1.2). They are generally numbered from

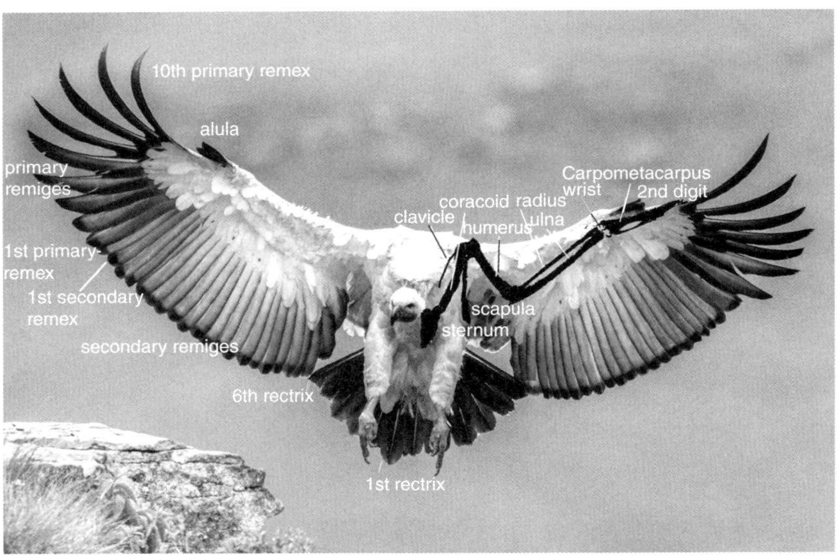

Fig. 1.1. Location and nomenclature of wing and tail feathers in the Cape vulture, *Gyps caprotheres*. The left wing shows the internal skeletal structure. Modified from Lingham-Soliar (2015).

the carpal joint to the end of the extended wing (descendent system) (Lingham-Soliar, 2015), although in some literature the primary feathers are numbered from the wing tip to the carpal joint (ascendant system).

The shorter secondary flight feathers grow from the ulna (forewing bone); these are always numbered from the carpal joint inwards towards the body. The innermost secondaries are also referred to as tertials or tertiaries, especially for passerine birds such as the raven (Proctor and Lynch, 1993). The primaries and secondaries together form the lifting surface of the wing.

The typical feather consists of a central shaft (rachis), applied to the portion of the axis of the feather that in life protrudes from the skin, and the lower part, which penetrates the skin and provides attachment and is termed the calamus or quill. Arising from the rachis are serial paired branches (barbs) extending out from the shaft at an angle and lying parallel to each other (Lingham-Soliar, 2017). The barbs possess further branches: the barbules. The barbules of adjacent barbs are attached to one another by hooks. The entire system comprising barbs and barbules forms a vane or web on either side of the rachis, providing the lifting surfaces of the wing and tail feathers. This construction ensures the elasticity of the feather web as well as the capacity of the barbs to re-establish linkage if the continuity of the web is interrupted (Fig. 1.2).

Feathers arise from the integument or skin of birds. The skin is fundamentally adapted to their life as active homeothermic (stable independent body temperature) animals. It is generally thin in areas covered by feathers and thick

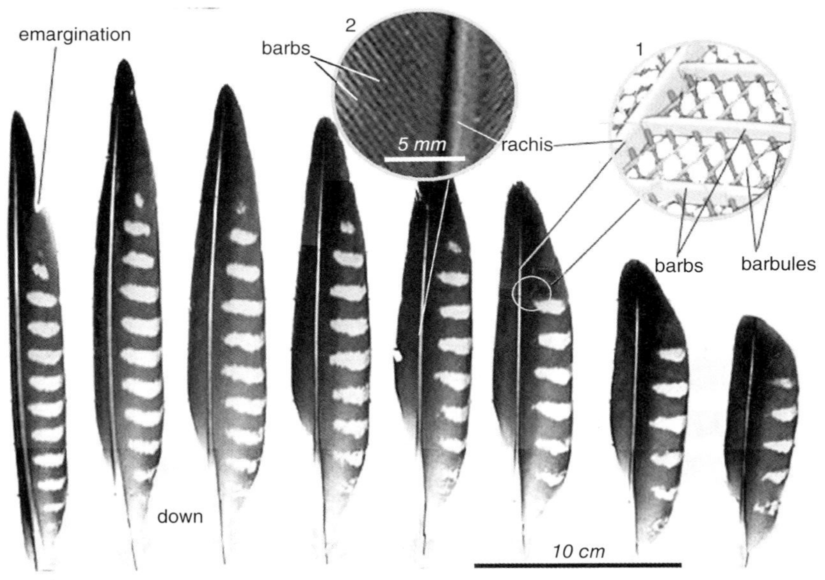

Fig. 1.2. Flight feathers in a juvenile peregrine falcon, *Falco peregrinus* (primaries 2 and 4 missing). The rachis is visible. Inset 1: diagrammatic view of rachis, barbs and barbules. Note that the sizes of the elements are not to scale. Inset 2: enlarged view showing relative sizes of rachis and barbs. Modified from Lingham-Soliar (2015).

in bare areas. Its germinative layer is like that in reptiles, but the corneous layer is much thinner in birds than in reptiles (Stettenheim, 2000), where in the latter it aids in protection.

Feathers are constructed of compact β-keratin, the keratin of reptiles and birds (sauropsids), a light rigid material (Fraser and Parry, 2008, 2011). The demands on the feather connected with flight are extraordinary: its qualities are almost paradoxical, having to be exceedingly light (or the bird would never leave the ground) and at the same time exceedingly tough to cope with the stresses of flight in which accelerations may reach extremely high g-forces (Clark, 2009). It is beyond the scope of this review to discuss the aerodynamics of bird flight but the reader may be interested in a review on flight in animals and some of the physics involved (Lingham-Soliar, 2015).

Recent research efforts using the microbes (fungus genus *Alternaria*) that normally parasitize bird feathers in the wild (Lingham-Soliar *et al.*, 2010) have now made it possible to attempt to answer the question that Gordon (1978) had posed many years ago. The unique assemblage of syncytial barbule fibres (SBFs) in the cortex of the rachis and barbs enabled a microstructure with a high 'work of fracture'. The model showed (Lingham-Soliar, 2014a) that rather than the traditional brick-and-mortar arrangement considered previously (Lingham-Soliar *et al.*, 2010), the architecture was more comparable with the 'brick-bridge-mortar' structure proposed for nacre (Song and Bai, 2001; Katti and Katti, 2006).

We know today that the fundamental structural component of the feather rachis is a system of continuous β-keratin SBFs that extend from the base of the rachis in a proximo-distal direction to its tip. Herein lies a problem if birds are to fly. The rachis may be described as a generalized cone of rapidly diminishing volume (Fig. 1.3).

Thus the volume of the cortex available for SBFs will decrease proximo-distally. Consequently, hundreds of SBFs in the rachidial cortex would theoretically have to be terminated before reaching the rachis tip – creating potentially thousands of inherently fatal crack-like defects. These defects of free ends or

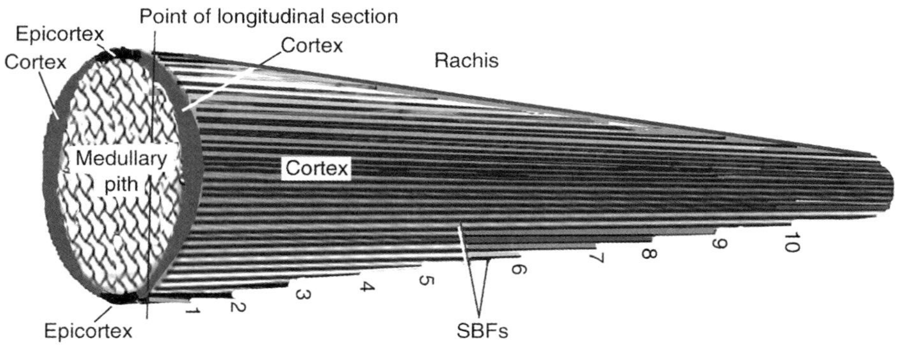

Fig. 1.3. Feather rachis as a cone. Diagrammatic view of the rachis as a tapering cone showing potential terminations of SBFs (numbered 1–10, along the edge for illustrative convenience) because of the linear decrease in cortex thickness in the proximo-distal direction. Modified from Lingham-Soliar (2017).

notches at numerous points of the cortex along the length of the rachis would locally concentrate the stress at each so-called notch (Lingham-Soliar, 2017). Simple mechanics shows that sudden failure in a material begins at a notch or crack that locally concentrates the stress. This is analogous to the scissor-snip a tailor makes before tearing a piece of fabric. Griffith (1921) showed that, according to thermodynamic principles, the magnitude of the stress concentration at a crack tip is dependent on the crack length, i.e. that the strain energy released in the area around the crack length is available for propagating the crack (similar to the scissor-snip). Given that there are thousands of SBFs in the feather, it is clear that there is a dangerous potential of numerous (hundreds of) self-perpetuating cracks in the feather cortex. The rachis of each feather would fail during the stresses of flight, resulting in a 'crash-and-burn' catastrophe. Clearly birds had solved the problem. The subject of the study (Lingham-Soliar, 2017) was: how? Briefly, for the first time we discovered that the SBFs of the barbs arise from well within the rachis, giving a stability hitherto unknown. This has not only solved the problem of the Griffith cracks but once again demonstrates the multifunctionality of bird structure in a unique tissue structure of the rachis that profoundly enhances the combined strength of the rachis and barbs.

FEATHERS AND PROTECTION

Two aspects of protection will be considered. The first is defence against predation and the second is protection from the environment.

It may be a chicken-and-egg question, i.e. which came first: protection or flight? The author's own view is that flight was the ultimate honing of a structure, the feather, which was evolving over 150 million years plus, from a basic component akin to the syncytial barbule filaments (Lingham-Soliar *et al.*, 2010). The syncytial barbule filaments were already equipped for a highly important function, thermoregulation (see below), which would later be vital to all aspects of bird life.

Even predatory birds such as hawks that prey on other birds in the air are aware of the ineffectiveness of their sharp talons and beak against the prey's protective densely feathered coat. Instead the hawk kills by diving and striking the bird in the back with its outstretched feet so as to impart a violent acceleration to the bird as a whole, which has the effect of breaking its neck (Gordon, 1978).

Bird feathers play another role during predation attempts that has evolved as a means of escape: birds often lose feathers because predators are more likely to grab feathers on the rump and the back than on the ventral side of an escaping bird. It is better that a predator (e.g. a cat) ends up with a mouthful of feathers than a mouthful of bird. Møller *et al.* (2006) predicted that 'the former feathers would have evolved to be relatively loosely attached as an antipredator strategy in species that frequently die from predation'.

The second part of this section considers how the feather has enabled birds to invade every form of environment on the planet. Many birds fly constantly in and out of trees and hedges and other obstacles, often using such cover as a refuge from their enemies. The unique structure of the feather vanes enables birds to get away with local scrapes and abrasions compared with the membranous wings of other active fliers, past and present.

The flat surface or vane of the pennaceous feather is deceptive and gives the impression of a continuous membrane. It was mentioned above that the barbs and barbules are central to the flight surface or venation of the pennaceous feather structure. Regal (1975) described how the interlocking barbules from adjacent barbs lock parts of the feather into a single tough, flat surface. The barbules of adjacent barbs are able to interlock essentially because those along the distal edge (edge away from the body) of a barb bear tiny hooklets that engage the unhooked (flange-bearing) barbules branching from the proximal edge (edge towards the body) of the adjacent barb. This is seen graphically in a scanning electron microscope (SEM) image of a barb (close to the rachis) in the peregrine falcon, *Falco peregrinus* (Fig. 1.4).

The system works like opposite pieces of Velcro and is as easily separated and reconnected. Thus, when forces are applied to the surface of this vane, part of the force will be absorbed in elastic deformation of the complex system, or if the force is too great the counterpart barbules will separate and either reattach

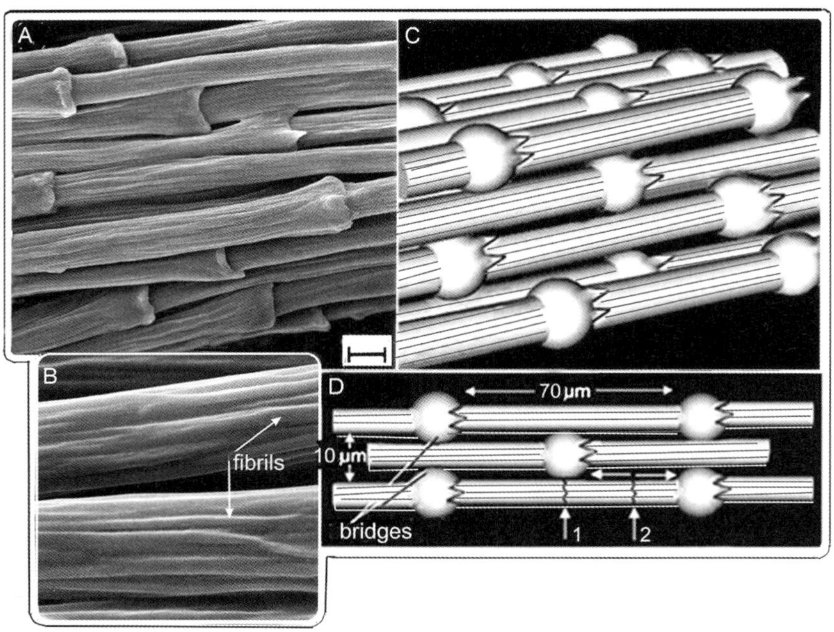

Fig. 1.4. Mechanical structure of syncytial barbule cells (fibres). (A) Syncytial barbule cells in the cortex of the feather rachis showing nodes. (B) Detail of the syncytial barbule cells comprising fibrils. (C) Diagrammatic representation of fibre bundling (syncytial barbules) in three dimensions. (D) Diagrammatic brick-bridge-mortar structure between syncytial barbules and polymer matrix demonstrating crack-stopping mechanisms (see text). Scale bar 5 µm. After Lingham-Soliar (2014c), courtesy of Springer, Heidelberg.

automatically, or if not, when the bird preens or nibbles its feathers, i.e. runs its beak along the separated barbules to reconnect them to the interlocked state. To put it simply, feathers avoid tears by having a structure that actually enables tearing but with the all-important differences: it occurs as part of a precise design and it is self-repairing or with a little attention from the bird.

This remarkable flight surface of feathers together with the formation into thick layers has enabled birds to live in densely structured habitats where even the loss of a reasonable number of feathers is a small price to pay for their ecological versatility. Besides, birds have one more 'ace up their sleeve'. When feathers may become too ragged for repair and inefficient, they are simply replaced. Most bird species moult their entire plumage at least once a year and in a few species twice.

THERMOREGULATION

All animals control their body temperature by a process known as thermoregulation, wherein the internal environment of the body is under the influence of both external and internal conditions. There are different ways in which terrestrial animals thermoregulate, such as behaviourally, by moving to a colder or warmer place, by activity to generate body heat, or by panting or sweating to lose it. They also thermoregulate physiologically, by activating internal metabolic processes that warm or cool the blood.

Today's mammals and birds have a high metabolism and are considered endotherms, which produce body heat internally. They possess biological temperature sensors that control heat production and switch on heat-loss mechanisms such as perspiration. Birds conserve body heat with specially constructed down feathers (Fig. 1.5).

Producing internal heat is one thing but it is an energetically expensive process and has to be conserved. Birds have to conserve their internally produced body heat and they do it uniquely, by growing feathers. Although all feathers are capable of both conserving or dissipating body heat in birds, this section considers the embryonic or down feathers and how they are specialized for insulation (Fig. 1.5).

The shape of down feathers is vital to their performance and primary purpose, which is to provide insulation. Down feathers form individual 'clumps' of more or less circular masses (as opposed to the flattened shape of flight feathers) that have a 'tree-like', highly organized self-similar structure (Yan and Wang, 2009), which is crucial to their thermal properties (Gao *et al.*, 2009). Each tree-like assemblage comprises a barb and branching barbules, described as primary and secondary structures, attached to the skin by a quill. The microstructure of barbs and barbules have been described in detail (Lingham-Soliar *et al.*, 2010; Lingham-Soliar and Murugan, 2013) and apply equally to the corresponding structures in down feathers.

Hooks (or hooklets) and nodes are vital features of the barbules of down feathers. To the author's knowledge, only the Silkie's down feather lacks hooklets (Feng *et al.*, 2014). These tiny hooks keep the barbules from becoming matted

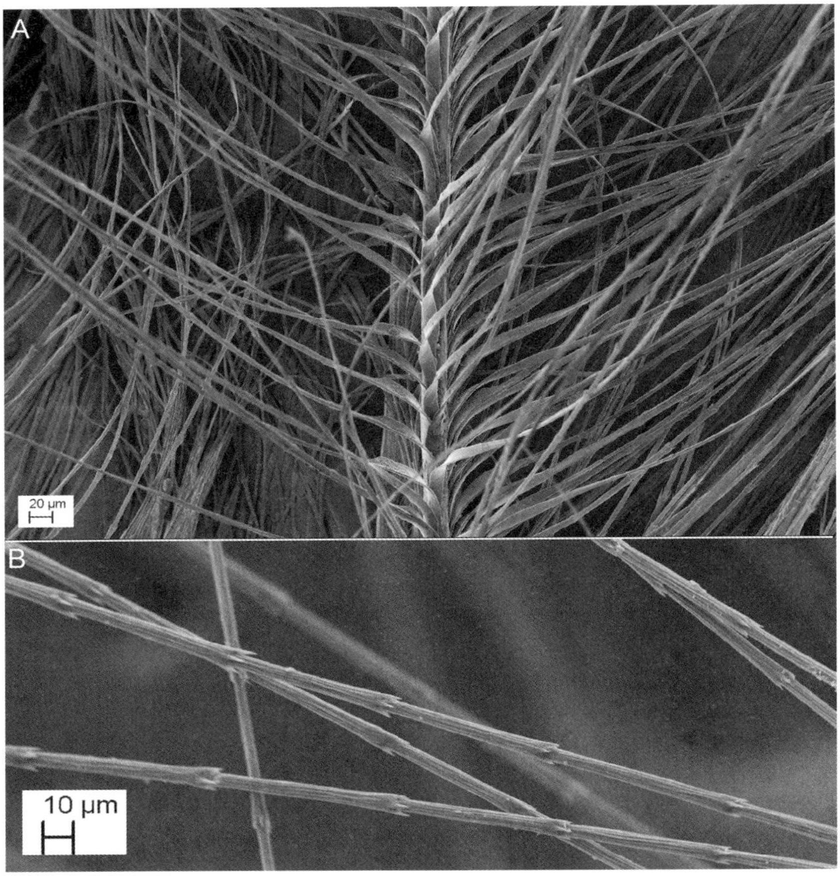

Fig. 1.5. Down feather, *Gallus gallus.* (A) Down feather showing barb and branching barbules. (B) Detail of the barbules. Some nodes lack (or have reduced) hooks, others have long hooks.

and flattened. In this way, the barbs and barbules remain fluffy, trapping air in the plumage for thermal insulation (Stettenheim, 2000). Of great importance too is the stiffness or Young's modulus of down feathers, especially with respect to the compressive resistance of each tree-like clump, i.e. it should retain its fluffy shape and avoid being compressed or, if compressed, possess enough elasticity to regain its former state. This compressive resistance is closely related to bending resistance and buckling resistance with respect to the microstructural properties of the rachis.

Continued research into the shape of the tree-like clumps, diameter of the barbs and structure of the nodes and hooks of the barbules in different birds is of considerable interest to multi-million-dollar industries involved in the manufacture of bedding and outdoor clothing. One of the problems in the use of downy feathers in the manufacture of outdoor wear is water resistance. Down feathers become ineffective in insulation and thermoregulation when wet or damp. This is immediately obvious in observations of chicks with wet down feathers, which may die rapidly from chill. Perhaps genetic manipulation to produce an ideal down feather will solve some of the problems in commercially utilized down feathers. Certainly more intensive research is called for with respect to down feather microstructure.

REFERENCES

Clark, C.J. (2009) Courtship dives of Anna's hummingbird offer insights into flight performance limits. *Proceedings of the Royal Society London B*. doi: 10.1098/rspb.2009.0508

Feng, C., Gao, Y., Dorshorst, B., Song, C., Xiaorong, G. *et al*. (2014) A cis-regulatory mutation of PDSS2 causes silky-feather in chickens. *PLOS Genetics* 10(8), e1004576. doi: 10.1371/journal.pgen.1004576

Fraser, R.D.B. and Parry, D.A.D. (2008) Molecular packing in the feather keratin filament . *Journal of Structural Biology* 162, 1–13. doi: 10.1016/j.jsb.2008.01.011.

Fraser, R.D.B. and Parry, D.A.D. (2011) The structural basis of the filament-matrix texture in the avian/reptilian group of hard b-keratins. *Journal of Structural Biology* 173, 391–405.

Gao, J., Pan, N. and Yu, W. (2009) Fractal character forecast of down fiber assembly microstructure. *Journal of Textile Institute* 100(6) 539–544. doi: 10.1080/00405000802055500

Gordon, J.E. (1978) *Structures*. Penguin, Harmondsworth, UK.

Griffith, A.A. (1921) The phenomena of rupture and flow in solids. *Philosophical Transactions of the Royal Society A (London)* 221, 163–198.

Katti, K.S and Katti, D.R. (2006) Why is nacre so tough and strong? *Material Science Engineering* 26, 1317–1324.

Lingham-Soliar, T. (2014a) Feather structure, biomechanics and biomimetics: the incredible lightness of being. *Journal of Ornithology* 155, 323–336. doi: 10.1007/s10336-013-1038-0.

Lingham-Soliar, T. (2014b) Response to comments by C. Palmer on my paper, Feather structure, biomechanics and biomimetics: the incredible lightness of being. Journal of Ornithology. doi: 10.1007/s10336-014-1093-1

Lingham-Soliar, T. (2014c) *The Vertebrate Integument, Volume 1*. Springer, Heidelberg, Germany.

Lingham-Soliar, T. (2015) *The Vertebrate Integument, Volume 2*. Springer, Heidelberg, Germany.

Lingham-Soliar, T. (2017) Microstructural tissue-engineering in the rachis and barbs of bird feathers. *Scientific Reports* 7, 45162. doi: 10.1038/srep45162.

Lingham-Soliar, T. and Murugan, N. (2013) A new helical crossed-fiber structure of β-keratin in flight feathers and its biomechanical implications. *PLOS ONE* 8, 1–12.

Lingham-Soliar, T., Bonser, R.H.C. and Wesley-Smith, J. (2010) Selective biodegradation of keratin matrix in feather rachis reveals classic bioengineering. *Proceedings of the Royal Society B: Biological Sciences* 277(1685), 1161–1168. doi: 10.1098/rspb.2009.1980.

Møller, A.P., Nielsen, J.T. and Erritzøe, J (2006) Losing the last feather: feather loss as an antipredator adaptation in birds. *Behavioral Ecology* 17, 1046–1056. doi: 10.1093/beheco/arl044

Proctor, N.S. and Lynch P.J. (1993) *Manual of Ornithology: Avian Structure and Function*. Yale University Press, New Haven, Connecticut.

Regal, P.J. (1975) The evolutionary origin of feathers. *The Quarterly Review of Biology* 50 (1), 35–66.

Song, F. and Bai, Y. (2001) Analysis of the strengthening and toughening of a biomaterial interface science. *China Series. Mathematics* 44(12), 1596–1601. doi: 10.1007/BF02880799

Stettenheim, P.R. (2000) The integumentary morphology of modern birds – an overview. *American Zoologist* 40, 461–477. doi: 10.1093/icb/40.4.461.

Yan, X. and Wang, Y. (2009) A feather and down category recognition system based on GA and SVM. *2009 International Conference on Education Technology and Computer*. IEEE Computer Society, Washington. Available at: http://ieeexplore.ieee.org/lpdocs/epic03/wrapper.htm?arnumber=5169466 (accessed 4 October 2018).

CHAPTER 2
Embryonic Development of the Avian Integument

Denis Headon*

The Roslin Institute and Royal (Dick) School of Veterinary Studies, University of Edinburgh, UK

ABSTRACT

The skin and its appendages, such as feathers and scales, form the interface between a bird and its environment. The size, number and distribution of feathers and the structure of the skin are defined during embryonic development through interactions between the dermal and epidermal tissues. A number of spontaneous mutations that alter feather distribution in the domestic chicken have been identified, defining key genes and intercellular signals that operate to determine their arrangement. This review summarizes the processes operating and structures formed during embryonic skin development in birds, and the origins of diversity in external appearance that arises from genetic variants acting in this period.

AVIAN SKIN STRUCTURE AND COMPONENTS

The avian skin functions as a barrier to water loss and infection, and in thermoregulation, display, camouflage and resistance to abrasion. As in other vertebrates, the skin is composed of an epithelium, called the epidermis, attached to a deeper connective tissue, called the dermis. The barrier functions of skin are largely carried out by the epidermis, which is a sheet of cells several layers thick. Most of the cells in the epidermis are keratinocytes, which adhere tightly to one another through cell–cell contacts and produce keratin to form a cytoskeleton. Adherens junctions and desmosomes fasten cells to one another, with the desmosomes connecting keratin cytoskeletons of adjacent cells to make a strong meshwork resistant to mechanical strain (Hatzfeld *et al.*, 2017). The proteins forming these junctions in chicken epidermis function in the same manner as

*denis.headon@roslin.ed.ac.uk

those in the skin of other vertebrates, including mammals, so that avian cells can readily attach to cells from species of different classes if cultured together (Mattey and Garrod, 1985). The cells at the base of the epidermis attach to a basement membrane, a very thin sheet of extracellular material that separates epidermis from dermis. The basal epidermal cells are those that divide, the cells departing the basement membrane stop dividing and instead mature to produce different keratins and lipids that will form the surface barrier. At the surface they lack nuclei and are shed continually and replenished by proliferation below. The epidermis sits atop and attached to the dermis, a connective tissue. This region is characterized by a substantial amount of extracellular material, particularly collagen fibres, and the predominant cells are the fibroblasts, which produce the connective tissue. The dermis carries the skin's blood vessels, lymphatics, nerves, fat and muscle (Pass, 1995; Stettenheim, 2000). This basic structure of the skin is dramatically altered to produce appendages: the feathers, scales, spurs, glands and the specialized skin of the beak and legs. Generally, in the appendages the epithelial component, derived from the epidermis, is the more active, either proliferating and keratinizing to make the feather or scale, or producing secretions in the case of the glands. The definition of which cells and regions will be set aside from the remainder of the skin to be modified into appendages occurs early in its development (Stettenheim, 2000) (Fig. 2.1).

The epidermis also hosts minority populations of melanocytes and dendritic antigen-presenting cells (Langerhans-like cells). Melanocytes are the designated cell type for production of melanin, which is transferred to other cell types for pigment colouration. An efficient repair of ultraviolet light-induced DNA damage in avian skin is achieved through the action of DNA photolyase enzymes, which are absent from mammals (Thoma, 1999), there is less requirement for melanin-based absorption of sunlight as a DNA protective mechanism in birds, so these pigments have free use in camouflage and display (Pass, 1995; Stettenheim, 2000). Chicken epidermis also carries antigen-presenting dendritic cells analogous to mammalian Langerhans cells (Perez-Torres and Ustarroz-Cano, 2001; Igyarto *et al.*, 2006), which act as immune sensors. These Langerhans-like cells can first appear in the epidermis prior to hatch, depending on breed and/or pathogen status, but they become much more numerous in the adult skin (Igyarto *et al.*, 2006).

This chapter aims to summarize the literature describing the origins of skin components and the basis for adult variation that arises from altered embryonic processes. As most experimental work has been done in the chicken, an experimental model used to understand skin development since the mid-20th century, the bulk of information is available from this species and that is reflected in this summary. Where distinct developmental processes occur in other species, these will be highlighted. Developmental ages of incubation given are for chicken, unless stated otherwise. Where primary literature has reported the timing of events in the embryo using embryonic stages, rather than time elapsed since lay, these have been converted here to days of incubation according to Hamburger and Hamilton (1951).

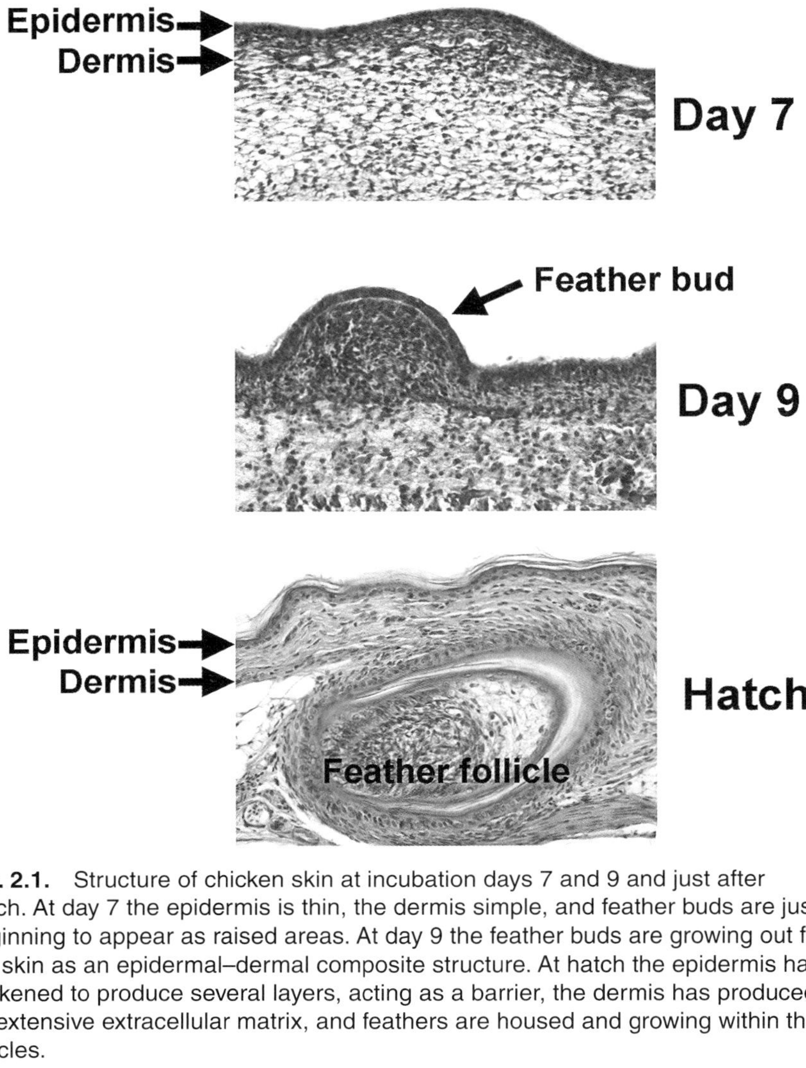

Fig. 2.1. Structure of chicken skin at incubation days 7 and 9 and just after hatch. At day 7 the epidermis is thin, the dermis simple, and feather buds are just beginning to appear as raised areas. At day 9 the feather buds are growing out from the skin as an epidermal–dermal composite structure. At hatch the epidermis has thickened to produce several layers, acting as a barrier, the dermis has produced an extensive extracellular matrix, and feathers are housed and growing within their follicles.

EMBRYONIC ORIGINS OF SKIN CELL TYPES

Though closely apposed and interacting throughout adult life, the different components of the skin have distinct origins in the embryo. The keratinocytes of the epidermis arise from the surface ectoderm, an epithelial sheet covering the chicken embryo from the first day of incubation (Bellairs and Osmond, 2005). The ectoderm is also the source of the central nervous system (brain and spinal cord). By day 6 of incubation the basal layer (the lowest epidermal layer, directly adjacent to the underlying dermis) is overlain by very flat cells forming a periderm (Parakkal and Matoltsy, 1968). This is a transient structure that serves as a barrier to the fluid surrounding the embryo until the epidermis proper has thickened to the point that it is capable of taking on this barrier role itself (Saathoff *et al.*, 2004). It is likely that, as in mammals, the periderm also serves in a Teflon-like capacity to prevent epidermal cells, which are tightly adherent to one another, from contacting and fusing different body parts together. This is exemplified in mammals by disorders of periderm formation, which lead to body sites close to one another, such as the limb and body wall of the trunk, becoming fused such that at birth they are enmeshed in a single web of skin (Richardson *et al.*, 2014). As the epidermis matures to produce its own upper cell layers as a barrier, the peridermal cells start to die from day 17 and the periderm is gone by hatch (Saathoff *et al.*, 2004).

The dermal cells of the skin have diverse origins, arising from distinct structures present in the early embryo. The dermis of the back of the trunk (the dorsum) arises from the somites, which are segmented blocks of tissue running along the body in pairs on either side of the forming spinal cord (called the neural tube). After appearing as tightly condensed balls of cells, the somites lose their compactness and give off migrating cells which contribute to the future trunk dermis, muscle and bone. Dermis towards the belly (ventral side) arises from the tissue still further to the sides of the somites, called the lateral plate mesoderm (Bellairs and Osmond, 2005).

At the most superficial part (the dorsal side) of the neural tube as it is forming, a special cell population called the neural crest is generated. These cells are highly migratory and form a range of different cell types as they disperse around the embryo, including in the skin the melanocytes that produce melanin pigment, Schwann cells that ensheathe peripheral nerves in myelin, and some dermal fibroblasts of the face and neck (Le Douarin *et al.*, 2004; Dupin *et al.*, 2006). In chicken, the melanocyte precursors arise and begin migrating between the second and third days of incubation, entering the skin about half a day later (Hulley *et al.*, 1991). The migration takes place starting from the midline on the back, where the cells are produced in the neural crest, across a peripheral route close to the embryo's surface (Thomas and Erickson, 2008). The melanocyte precursors transit slowly through the dermis upon entering the skin, most of them eventually populating the epidermis and then entering the feathers and their follicles as these develop. In the chicken embryo the onset of melanin pigment production in the skin is breed specific, but can occur as early as day 5 of incubation (Hulley *et al.*, 1991). These embryonic events populate the skin with melanocytes, setting the scene for the many colour variations that are apparent in mature birds.

A change in the embryonic trajectory and proliferation of the migrating melanocyte precursors (called melanoblasts) occurs in the Silkie breed due to a mutation that increases the expression of the *EDN3* gene (Dorshorst *et al.*, 2011; Shinomiya *et al.*, 2012). An additional cell migration route down into the embryo's body, as well as the normal spreading of these cells across the body close to the skin surface (Faraco *et al.*, 2001), causes melanocytes to accumulate and persist lifelong in the internal tissues as well as in the dermis (Ortolani-Machado *et al.*, 2008). These altered embryonic events seed the internal organs with melanocytes, which persist lifelong in connective tissue and produce the characteristic dark flesh (fibromelanosis) of the Silkie and some other traditional breeds. In the White Leghorn the melanocyte precursors enter the skin and feathers, but are susceptible to cell death once they begin to produce pigment (Jimbow *et al.*, 1974). The major effect locus causing this melanocyte loss is a mutation in *PMEL17*, which encodes a protein involved in the production and cellular packaging of melanin pigment (Kerje *et al.*, 2004).

Along the body of the embryo a systematic ordering of HOX gene expression is laid down at early stages. These genes encode a set of related transcription factors that regulate gene expression in a manner that defines a cell's position along the head-to-tail (anterior–posterior) axis of the animal. A transcription factor is a protein that binds to specific DNA sequences, controlling the expression of genes near that binding site by either increasing or decreasing their rate of synthesis. The HOX genes are so called as their mutation leads to homeotic transformations, in which a body part is found in the incorrect location along the head-to-tail axis of the body. The HOX genes have served as a unifying principle in developmental biology, as they are found in all bilaterian animals and are expressed in the same order along the length of the body. This order matches the arrangement of the genes in their clusters in the genome, such that the genes located early in a cluster (which are designated with low numbers) are active towards the head of the embryo, while those further along a cluster (designated with sequentially higher numbers, up to 13) become active further along the body towards the tail. In insects only a single cluster is present, while this has been expanded to four clusters in the vertebrates, where they are labelled from A through D. The HOX expression profile at a given location can be thought of as a ZIP or postal code, defining for a cell where in the body it lies relative to head and tail, and therefore what type of structure it should cooperate with its neighbouring cells to develop into (Pick, 2016). The embryonic skin maintains a distinct graded profile of HOX gene expression (Johansson and Headon, 2014), with impacts on regional identity of skin and its appendages (see below).

EVENTS IN EARLY FEATHER BUD FORMATION

During the course of its development the skin is modified in specific areas to produce appendages, such as scales, feathers, glands, combs and wattles. Feathers are the most prominent and numerous skin appendage, comprising about 6% of the average adult bird's weight (Stettenheim, 2000). The feather itself is generated by the epidermis, and is generated by and retained in a follicle that is largely epidermal, but at its base having input from the dermis which contributes the dermal papilla and pulp (Yu *et al.*, 2004).

The feathers are present in tracts of stereotypical location, most of which are present bilaterally, arranged around or on the limbs (humeral, femoral, alar, crural) or on the breast (ventral). Some tracts form along the middle of the back and are present as single tracts (capital, spinal, caudal). Each tract is defined in the embryo by a distinct site of initiation (or bilaterally paired sites of initiation), most becoming first detectable by day 6 of incubation in chicken by streaks of expression of specific genes, such as *CTNNB1* (Fig. 2.2). These streaks are underlain by a dermis that is more densely cellular (i.e. the cells are more numerous and

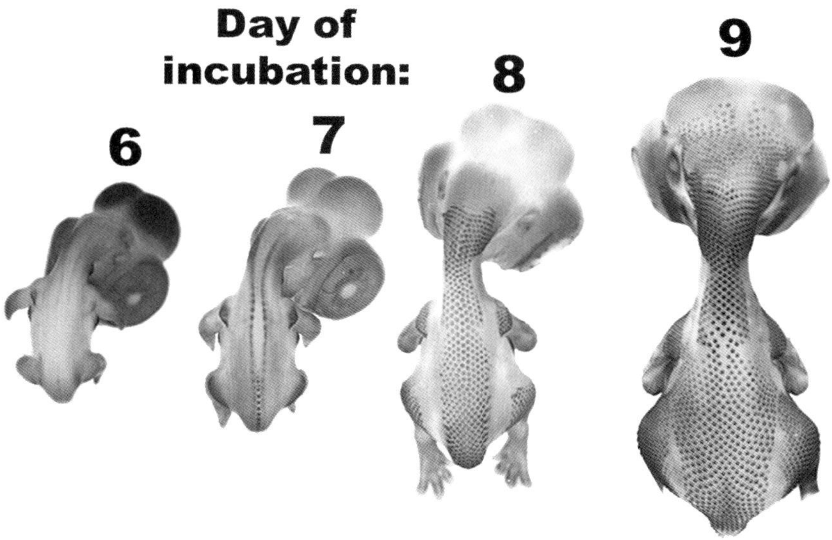

Fig. 2.2. The process of feather formation at different stages of chicken embryonic development. Areas of skin beginning to form a feather are visible as dots, here revealed by detection of mRNA from the *CTNNB1* gene. The feather tracts appear first as stripes, which break up and spread across the skin, leaving rows of feather primordia in their wake.

hence closer together) than non-tract skin. These streaks quickly break up into a row of spots, each of these spots being a cluster of cells that begins rapid outgrowth to form a bud, which first becomes externally visible as a raised dome in chicken embryos soon after its formation (Fonseca *et al.*, 2013) (Fig. 2.1). The bud is composed of more tightly packed epidermal cells, called a placode, and underlying this is a compacted mass of dermal cells, called the dermal condensate. Prior to splitting into buds, the initial streaks of gene expression expand outwards, followed by addition of further rows of feather buds every few hours (about 7 h for addition of paired rows in the chicken spinal tract). The spreading waves do not collide laterally, such that most tracts do not merge but instead leave down-feathered or non-feathered (apteric) regions between them. The tracts along the head-to-tail axis, the capital, spinal and caudal, do meet to yield a continuous feather covering from head to tail. The tracts are similar in position between avian species, though their relative sizes and boundaries are not (Clench, 1970).

Large birds generally have many more feathers than small birds, with swans carrying more than 25,000 feathers (Ammann, 1937) and a hummingbird fewer than 1000 (Wetmore, 1936). This difference is in part influenced by differing skin area and body proportions, but a major effect on the number of feathers carried by birds also depends on whether they develop secondary feathers or not. In the chicken, new feathers are produced only at the leading edges of the tract waves, without later addition of feathers between the existing primary ones. However, in birds with extensive down feathers, such as ducks and geese, a later process of insertion of secondary feathers occurs after the primary feathers have formed. In the duck, the primary feathers form in a wave, much as in chicken – though not on the neck – from E8, completing the tracts at E11. The secondary follicles then begin to form over the entire body, including tract, apterium and neck, and do so not in rows following a wave, but in a more haphazard manner (Fig. 2.3). In the goose the primary feathers are reported to be detectable as extending buds from day 14 of incubation, and the more numerous and smaller secondary feathers from day 18 onwards (Wu *et al.*, 2008).

PROGRESSION FROM FEATHER BUD TO FEATHER FOLLICLE

Each feather bud, beginning to be visible from day 7 of incubation, grows outwards rapidly to form an extending filament. As they extend, the filaments orient their tips towards the embryo's tail, becoming angled along the body. Early growth of the buds occurs through cell proliferation at their tips, but the growth zone of the feather steadily shifts towards the base, which then serves as the site of cell production, and thus feather growth, through life (Chodankar *et al.*, 2003). By day 11 of incubation the epidermis at the base of the growing filament descends into the underlying dermis as a ring around the feather to make the permanent follicle (Pass, 1995) that produces and houses the feathers. Within the extending filament antagonistic interactions between cellular signals resolve themselves into threads of cells destined to die through programmed cell death (apoptosis), releasing separated strands. If these strands are parallel to one another and run straight down the filament towards the skin surface, as in chicken embryos, then a simple down feather with no central stalk or rachis is formed. If, as in duck embryos, these strands curve around the filament as they run down, forming a helix, then they attach to a region on one side of the growing filament, which forms the rachis (Yu *et al.*, 2004; Harris *et al.*, 2005).

FEATHER ARRANGEMENT AND ITS UNDERLYING CELLULAR AND MOLECULAR CONTROLS

Within the tracts the feather buds appear spaced apart at equal distances from one another in a regular pattern. Each of these locations of future feather budding is marked out from the surrounding skin by a tighter packing of epidermis and underneath a clumping of dermal cells, drawn together through the collagen-rich extracellular matrix. Experimental separation of epidermis from dermis has been used to show that both layers must be in contact to form feathers; neither will do so if maintained in isolation. Reassembling separated epidermis and dermis in new combinations revealed that a high cell density in the dermis is required for feather formation, and that epidermis from essentially any region of the skin will respond to sitting atop a dense, highly cellular dermis by producing feathers (Johansson and Headon, 2014).

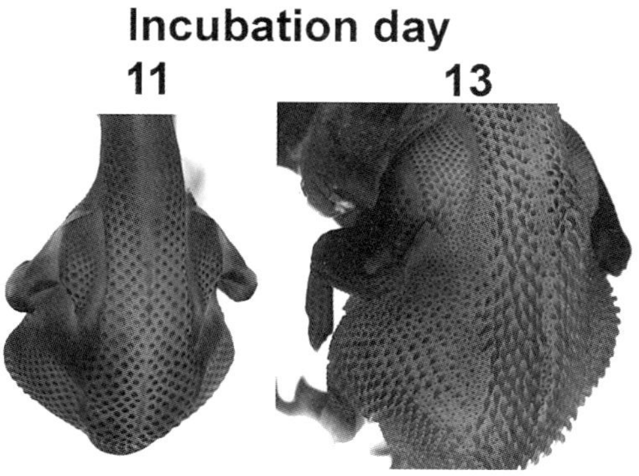

Fig. 2.3. Primary and secondary feather bud formation in duck embryos (visualized by detection of *CTNNB1* mRNA). At incubation day 11 the tract feathers have formed in rows. By day 13 these primary feathers have grown longer and secondary feather buds are appearing as small dots across the entire skin.

The regular arrangement of feather buds has attracted the interest of theoreticians curious about the general mechanisms underlying biological pattern formation and an extensive literature suggesting the basis for this spacing arrangement has been established. The reaction–diffusion theory, originating from Alan Turing's ideas, suggests that cells signal to one another with conflicting feather-promoting and inhibitory signals to define the locations at which the feathers will form, following which moving cells act according to these instructions. Alternative mechanisms for cellular rearrangement to make a feather, based on physical forces in the tissue or cell movement, have also been proposed (Painter *et al.*, 2012). These systems of organizing repeating patterns are quite different to that conferred by the HOX genes mentioned above, which apply a precise spatial coordinate to each location. These systems for making repeated patterns, like those of the feathers, can be best thought of as local groups of cells following the simple rule: 'if there is no feather bud nearby then we will develop into a feather ourselves – and prevent our neighbours from doing so'.

Experimental understanding of the mechanism underlying initiation of feather development was boosted by the appearance of the 'scaleless' mutant in the 1950s (Abbott and Asmundson, 1957). On an appropriate genetic background, homozygous scaleless individuals lack scales, spurs and feathers. This mutant has been used for decades as an experimental model in which neither epidermal placodes nor dermal condensates characteristic of feather formation appear during development, other than for the occasional 'escaping' feather (Houghton *et al.*, 2007). Embryonic tissue recombination experiments showed that the defect in this mutant lies within the epidermis, as scaleless mutant epidermis combined with normal dermis fails to form feathers, while the reciprocal combination does undergo feather development. This established a crucial active role for epidermis in the process of feather and scale initiation, rather than simply a passive following of dermal instructions (Sengel and Abbott, 1963). The scaleless line has also been used to assess the importance of feathers in avian behaviour (revealing that birds dust bathe even without a plumage to clean) (Vestergaard *et al.*, 1999), adult physiology (in large-bodied broiler chickens feathers prove to be a major impediment to heat loss and therefore health and growth) (Azoulay *et al.*, 2011) and in detecting competition between growing feathers and other organ systems for resources prior to hatching (Hadad *et al.*, 2014). The causative mutation in scaleless has been identified as a disruption of the fibroblast growth factor 20 gene (*FGF20*) (Wells *et al.*, 2012). Fibroblast growth factors are a large family of related proteins with many roles in organ development, originally identified based on their effects on fibroblast growth. These proteins are released from their cell of production and can diffuse through the extracellular space to bind to highly specific receptors on neighbouring cells, changing the behaviour or state of the receiving cell.

By the time of identification of the causative mutation in scaleless, the FGF family, together with other important signals that operate in a conceptually similar manner, had already been implicated in feather development. Most of these factors were identified from candidate studies focusing on conserved cellular signals found across the animal kingdom. These include the bone morphogenetic protein (BMP) family as inhibitors of feather development (Jung *et al.*, 1998; Noramly and Morgan, 1998), FGF family (Widelitz *et al.*, 1996) and tumour growth factor β (TGFβ) family (Ting-Berreth and Chuong, 1996) as attractors of cells, and the wingless/INT (WNT) class as general modulators of feather development (Chang *et al.*, 2004). The precise roles of these proteins in defining which cells become feather and which do not, which specific family members of each class are relevant, and how these pathways interact with one another, remain under investigation (Painter *et al.*, 2012). Harder to study, and largely hidden from genetic approaches, has been a possible role for physical forces in feather development. Though suggested as a means to generate feather patterns some decades ago (Oster *et al.*, 1983; Bard, 1990), consideration of such influences has languished compared with the many studies focused on molecular signals. However, a role for physical forces in influencing molecular signalling has recently been defined in developing chicken skin (Shyer *et al.*, 2017), emerging as an integration between signal-based and mechanical-based modes of development.

VARIATIONS IN REGIONAL FEATHER ARRANGEMENT

Some individual genetic variants with major effects on feather distribution have been identified and selectively bred, generally for their aesthetic interest and as curiosities. The 'Muffs and Beard' (Mb) and the 'Crest' (Cr) traits are each caused by a single dominant gene, and each is characterized by the presence of longer than typical feathers on top of the head (Cr) or under the beak and neck (Mb). The Mb trait was shown to be caused by a rearrangement including duplication of *HOXB7* and *HOXB8* at the HOXB cluster on chromosome 27, leading to expression of *HOXB8* in the chin and neck region (Guo *et al.*, 2016). Similarly, the Crest trait was mapped to the HOXC cluster and found to be associated with expression of the *HOXC8* gene in the embryonic head skin (Wang *et al.*, 2012). *HOXB8* and *HOXC8* are 'high number' HOX genes that are located far down their respective HOX gene array in the genome and thus are normally active more towards the tail, on the trunk of the embryo. Activation of these genes on the top of the head, or under the beak and neck, alters the developmental behaviour of the skin in these regions, partly transforming it to the trunk identity, which is characterized by growth of longer feathers. The HOX genes were originally identified as being the cause of homeotic transformations in insects, such as legs growing in place of antennae. Though not as dramatic, these old chicken varieties echo in the skin the large-scale homeotic transformations observed in insects that served to advance developmental genetics in the 20th century (Pick, 2016).

A distinct type of crest has been identified in the domestic pigeon, where a crest phenotype is defined not by the presence of longer feathers on the top of the head, but instead by a 180° inversion of feather orientation solely on the neck so that the tips point towards the head instead of the tail. This causes a flaring presentation of the feathers around the head, akin to that of a protective cone used after veterinary surgery. In pigeons this trait is caused by a mutation in *EPHB2* (Shapiro *et al.*, 2013), which encodes a protein that controls signalling and senses cell-to-cell contacts. Strikingly, an exactly analogous phenotype in the ringneck dove is also caused by a mutation in *EPHB2*, though at a different site in the gene (Vickrey *et al.*, 2015). The flipping of feather orientation is readily apparent as the feather buds first appear and begin to grow in the embryos of these crested birds (Shapiro *et al.*, 2013), but why the effect is confined to the neck is unknown.

Regional variation in feather distribution is also apparent in the 'Naked neck' (*Na*) chicken, a trait widely dispersed across the globe in village and production lines (Merat, 1986). This trait is caused by a single co-dominant locus and is characterized by absence of feathers on the neck, though they remain on the crown of the head, and reduced tract width on the body that is not usually apparent due to coverage of the skin with the feathers that remain (Crawford, 1976). Homozygous *Na* chickens have a total feather reduction of about 40%, while heterozygotes have a reduction of 20% from wild type and also a tuft or bib of feathers at the base of the neck that distinguishes them from homozygotes (Singh *et al.*, 2001). This trait is associated with increased agricultural production in hot conditions (Merat, 1986; Yalcin *et al.*, 1997; Deeb and Cahaner, 2001; Singh *et al.*, 2001; Adomako *et al.*, 2014) and was mapped to chromosome 3 (Pitel *et al.*, 2000). Fine mapping of the mutation led to its identification as insertion of a segment of DNA from chromosome 1 into a gene-free region of chromosome 3. This insertion leads to increased production of a nearby gene, *BMP12* (also called *GDF7*) (Mou *et al.*, 2011), belonging to the BMP class of molecules previously defined as inhibitors of feather formation (Jung *et al.*, 1998; Noramly and Morgan, 1998). However, the reason for the regional selectivity of feather suppression by increased production of *BMP12* was not immediately clear from these earlier studies. Further experiments on cultured embryonic skin revealed that different parts of the skin have intrinsically different sensitivities to BMP, such that the neck and also the margins of the tracts are more sensitive than the centre regions of the tracts. On the neck this relates to the presence of retinoic acid, a biologically active metabolite of vitamin A (retinol) which serves as a signal that enhances BMP's effects in suppressing feather formation. This underlying 'map' of BMP sensitivity appears to be present in many bird species, but requires shifting BMP levels to be revealed as an altered feather arrangement (Mou *et al.*, 2011). The basis for the selective production of retinoic acid on the neck is unknown, but may ultimately rest on regulation by the HOX genes already mentioned. These findings indicate that genetically reducing feather number is a process that respects unseen gradations and distinctions between regions of the embryonic skin.

DEVELOPMENT AND VARIATIONS OF FOOT SKIN

Foot skin is distinguished from that of the body by being scaled, in most birds, with large rectangular scutes on the dorsal (top of the foot, when adult) surface and smaller circular reticulate scales on the ventral (underside) contact surface (Stettenheim, 2000). The development of scutate scales begins from day 10 of incubation in the chicken and is detectable using many of the same marker genes as those that reveal early feather development (Fig. 2.4). The epidermis at these locations specified to become scale undergoes a transient halt in proliferation, forms a placode, and thickens to keratinize, though without the prominent dermal condensation that accompanies the placode in feather development (Sawyer and Knapp, 2003).

That scales and feathers have a similar genetic basis for their formation is apparent from the activity of many of the same genes in the development of both types of structure, and underscored by the fact that the scaleless mutant lacks both feathers and scales. Indeed, foot skin can quite readily switch to producing feathers rather than scales, as seen in a number of species of wild and domesticated birds with feathered feet. Experimentally, a number of different manipulations applied to change the signals in the developing foot are capable of triggering a change to feather rather than scale formation. These include the already mentioned BMP (Zou and Niswander, 1996), retinoic acid (Dhouailly, 1983) and WNT (Widelitz *et al.*, 2000) molecular pathways. This facility of switching to feathered feet is also attested by the number of different mutations that cause feathered feet, termed ptilopody (Somes, 1992). Though progress has been made

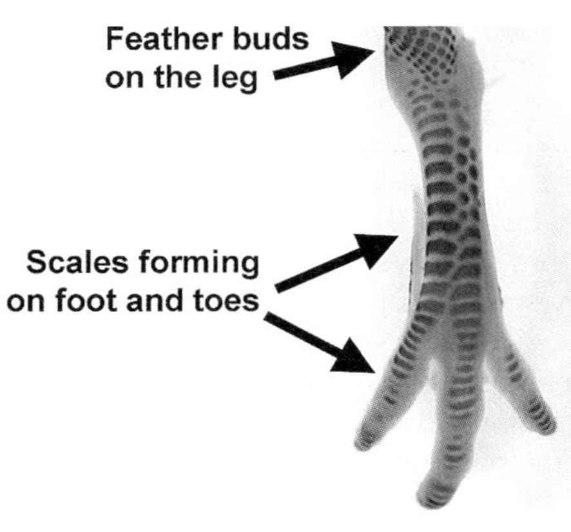

Fig. 2.4. The beginning of scale development on a chicken foot at incubation day 10. The areas of skin destined to form scales are emerging as approximately rectangular plates, revealed here by detection of *CTNNB1* mRNA.

in mapping the somewhat complex genetics of ptilopody in chicken (Dorshorst *et al.*, 2010; Sun *et al.*, 2015), the molecular basis for feathered feet in the domestic pigeon has to date been better characterized and leads the way in understanding the developmental origin of this phenomenon. In the pigeon, feathered feet arise from mutations that lead to altered expression of specific transcription factors that define leg (hindlimb) versus wing (forelimb) identity. One of these, *TBX5*, is normally expressed in the wing, but due to mutation becomes active in the leg as well. A second mutation that also causes ptilopody is characterized by reduced expression of the *PITX1* gene in the leg. *PITX1* normally promotes the development of hindlimb structural features, as opposed to forelimb features. These changes in gene expression, either in isolation or in combination, cause the skin of the leg to take on characteristics of the wing, and so produce feathers in place of scales. The changes to the skin are accompanied by some alterations in soft tissues, with tendon insertion sites and muscle orientation in the leg being somewhat modified. Examination of chicken embryos with ptilopody has revealed the expression of *TBX5* in the leg and thus in chicken as in pigeon the effect is to change the leg skin cells' identity to that of wing, though the ultimate genetic trigger for this is not understood (Domyan *et al.*, 2016). It is likely that the altered activity of these two transcription factors changes the production of intercellular signals, thereby diverting cells from constructing scales to producing feathers.

DEVELOPMENT AND VARIATIONS OF HEAD SKIN

In addition to its feathers, the head carries unique structures and modifications of the skin. In chicken the beak appears in the embryo at day 5 of incubation and a projection at its tip recognized as the egg tooth becomes apparent on day 6 (Hamburger and Hamilton, 1951) or day 8 (Fonseca *et al.*, 2013). The beak becomes covered with a specialized integument, termed the rhamphotheca, which is typically hard and highly keratinized (Stettenheim, 2000). The beak's internal structure is of bone, with great variety of form apparent in the natural world, serving as a prime example and inspiration in evolutionary biology. Such variation in beak shape has been linked to changes in BMP signalling processes (Abzhanov *et al.*, 2004; Wu *et al.*, 2004) and a major contribution to the distinction between blunt versus pointed beaks in Galapagos finches has been ascribed to variation at the *ALX1* gene (Lamichhaney *et al.*, 2015).

A variety of combs and wattles are found on birds, including the domestic chicken. The comb is the most prominent and most obviously variable of these in the chicken. Combs first appear at days 6–7 of incubation (Bellairs and Osmond, 2005) as a ridge lying between the eyes, just behind the beak. This grows a small amount, with the overall shape being determined in the embryo. The comb is based around a dermis of unusual structure, with extensive collagen fibres and hyaluronic acid, which binds to water and swells, giving a plump appearance. The red colour comes from blood visible in a capillary network just under the skin. At hatch, male and female combs are the same small size, the later growth to adulthood coming under major influence of testosterone (Hardesty, 1931; Ludwig and Boas, 1950).

Several variant forms of the comb exist, with their inheritance patterns and interactions used as a model in the early history of vertebrate genetics. Whereas the wild-type comb is a single tall serrated blade, the Pea comb projects less from the head (often as three knobbed ridges); the Rose comb is broad with many projections; while duplex combs are either fully duplicated rather normal combs or else paired tubular growths akin to fleshy horns. In recent years the precise molecular genetic basis for these different comb shapes has been defined. All three of these comb variants are caused by large structural mutations leading to production of a transcription factor in comb skin that is not normally expressed there. Pea comb affects *SOX5* (Wright *et al.*, 2009), Rose comb affects *MNR2* (Imsland *et al.*, 2012) and duplex combs *EOMES* (Dorshorst *et al.*, 2014). Together these mutations reveal a surprising commonality between the basis for each of these changes to comb form (Headon, 2015). Further developmental studies have found that the Pea comb mutation influences comb shape through suppression of signalling from the protein growth factor SHH (Boije *et al.*, 2012), beginning to shed light on how different morphological routes are achieved by these genetic variants.

CONCLUSION

The skin of birds develops in a similar manner to that of other land-living vertebrates, with an epidermis and dermis assembling early, and peridermal protection operating until the epidermis has matured sufficiently to act as barrier. The dermis has more diverse embryonic origins than the epidermis. The production of appendages relies on interaction between the skin's epidermal and dermal components, using a range of signals and with input from physical processes, influenced at different sites by an underlying molecular code that defines location-specific characteristics. Though there are important growth processes taking place before and after, the events critical in defining the number and distribution of appendages, and so much of the external appearance of a bird, take place in chicken between incubation days 5 and 11. With its rich history, recent discoveries and new genetic tools, chicken will continue as a leading model system in developmental biology, as well as a key production animal in global agriculture.

REFERENCES

Abbott, U. and Asmundson, V. (1957) Scaleless, an inherited ectodermal defect in the domestic fowl. *Journal of Heredity* 48, 63–70.

Abzhanov, A., Protas, M., Grant, B.R., Grant, P.R. and Tabin, C.J. (2004) Bmp4 and morphological variation of beaks in Darwin's finches. *Science* 305, 1462–1465.

Adomako, K., Olympio, O.S., Hagan, J.K. and Hamidu, J.A. (2014) Growth performance of crossbred naked neck and normal feathered laying hens kept in tropical villages. *British Poultry Science* 55, 701–708.

Ammann, G.A. (1937) Number of contour feathers of Cygnus and Xanthocephalus. *The Auk* 54, 201–202.

Azoulay, Y., Druyan, S., Yadgary, L., Hadad, Y. and Cahaner, A. (2011) The viability and performance under hot conditions of featherless broilers versus fully feathered broilers. *Poultry Science* 90, 19–29.

Bard, J.B. (1990) Traction and the formation of mesenchymal condensations in vivo. *Bioessays* 12, 389–395.

Bellairs, R. and Osmond, M. (2005) *The Atlas of Chick Development*, 2nd edn. Elsevier Academic Press, London.

Boije, H., Harun-Or-Rashid, M., Lee, Y.J., Imsland, F., Bruneau, N. *et al.* (2012) Sonic Hedgehog-signalling patterns the developing chicken comb as revealed by exploration of the pea-comb mutation. *PLOS ONE* 7, e50890.

Chang, C.H., Jiang, T.X., Lin, C.M., Burrus, L.W., Chuong, C.M. *et al.* (2004) Distinct Wnt members regulate the hierarchical morphogenesis of skin regions (spinal tract) and individual feathers. *Mechanisms of Development* 121, 157–171.

Chodankar, R., Chang, C.H., Yue, Z., Jiang, T.X., Suksaweang, S. *et al.* (2003) Shift of localized growth zones contributes to skin appendage morphogenesis: role of the Wnt/beta-catenin pathway. *Journal of Investigative Dermatology* 120, 20–26.

Clench, M.H. (1970) Variability in body pterylosis, with special reference to genus Passer. *The Auk* 87, 650–691.

Crawford, R.D. (1976) Incomplete dominance of gene for naked neck in domestic fowl. *Poultry Science* 55, 820–822.

Deeb, N. and Cahaner, A. (2001) Genotype-by-environment interaction with broiler genotypes differing in growth rate. 1. The effects of high ambient temperature and naked-neck genotype on lines differing in genetic background. *Poultry Science* 80, 695–702.

Dhouailly, D. (1983) Early events in retinoic acid-induced ptilopody in the chick embryo. *Wilhelm Roux's Archives of Developmental Biology* 192, 21–27.

Domyan, E.T., Kronenberg, Z., Infante, C. R., Vickrey, A.I., Stringham, S.A. *et al.* (2016) Molecular shifts in limb identity underlie development of feathered feet in two domestic avian species. *Elife* 5, e12115. doi: 10.7554/eLife.12115.

Dorshorst, B., Okimoto, R. and Ashwell, C. (2010) Genomic regions associated with dermal hyperpigmentation, polydactyly and other morphological traits in the Silkie chicken. *Journal of Heredity* 101, 339–350.

Dorshorst, B., Molin, A.M., Rubin, C.J., Johansson, A.M., Stromstedt, L. *et al.* (2011) A complex genomic rearrangement involving the endothelin 3 locus causes dermal hyperpigmentation in the chicken. *PLOS Genetics* 7, e1002412.

Dorshorst, B., Harun-Or-Rashid, M., Bagherpoor, A.J., Rubin, C.J., Ashwell, C. *et al.* (2014) A genomic duplication is associated with ectopic eomesodermin expression in the embryonic chicken comb and two duplex-comb phenotypes. *PLOS Genetics* 11, e1004947.

Dupin, E., Creuzet, S. and Le Douarin, N.M. (2006) The contribution of the neural crest to the vertebrate body. *Advances in Experimental Medicine and Biology* 589, 96–119.

Faraco, C.D., Vaz, S.A., Pastor, M.V. and Erickson, C.A. (2001) Hyperpigmentation in the Silkie fowl correlates with abnormal migration of fate-restricted melanoblasts and loss of environmental barrier molecules. *Developmental Dynamics* 220, 212–225.

Fonseca, E.T., Silva, F.M.D., Alcantara, D., Cardoso, R.C., Franciolli, A.L. *et al.* (2013) Embryonic development of chicken (*Gallus gallus domesticus*) from 1st to 19th day – ectodermal structures. *Microscopy Research and Technique* 76, 1217–1225.

Guo, Y., Gu, X., Sheng, Z., Wang, Y., Luo, C. *et al.* (2016) A complex structural variation on chromosome 27 leads to the ectopic expression of HOXB8 and the Muffs and beard phenotype in chickens. *PLOS Genetics* 12, e1006071.

Hadad, Y., Cahaner, A. and Halevy, O. (2014) Featherless and feathered broilers under control versus hot conditions. 2. Breast muscle development and growth in pre- and posthatch periods. *Poultry Science* 93, 1076–1088.

Hamburger, V. and Hamilton, H.L. (1951) A series of normal stages in the development of the chick embryo. *Journal of Morphology* 88, 49–92.

Hardesty, M. (1931) The structural basis for the response of the comb of the Brown Leghorn fowl to the sex hormones. *American Journal of Anatomy* 47, 277–323.

Harris, M.P., Williamson, S., Fallon, J.F., Meinhardt, H. and Prum, R.O. (2005) Molecular evidence for an activator-inhibitor mechanism in development of embryonic feather branching. *Proceedings of the National Academy of Sciences of the United States of America* 102, 11734–11739.

Hatzfeld, M., Keil, R. and Magin, T.M. (2017) Desmosomes and intermediate filaments: their consequences for tissue mechanics. *Cold Spring Harbor Perspectives in Biology* 9(6), a029157.

Headon, D. (2015) Morphological mutations: lessons from the cockscomb. *PLOS Genetics* 11, e1004979.

Houghton, L., Lindon, C.M., Freeman, A. and Morgan, B.A. (2007) Abortive placode formation in the feather tract of the scaleless chicken embryo. *Developmental Dynamics* 236, 3020–3030.

Hulley, P.A., Stander, C.S. and Kidson, S.H. (1991) Terminal migration and early differentiation of melanocytes in embryonic chick skin. *Developmental Biology* 145, 182–194.

Igyarto, B.Z., Lacko, E., Olah, I. and Magyar, A. (2006) Characterization of chicken epidermal dendritic cells. *Immunology* 119, 278–288.

Imsland, F., Feng, C., Boije, H., Bed'hom, B., Fillon, V. *et al.* (2012) The Rose-comb mutation in chickens constitutes a structural rearrangement causing both altered comb morphology and defective sperm motility. *PLOS Genetics* 8, e1002775.

Jimbow, K., Szabo, G. and Fitzpatrick, T.B. (1974) Ultrastructural investigation of autophagocytosis of melanosomes and programmed death of melanocytes in White Leghorn feathers: a study of morphogenetic events leading to hypomelanosis. *Developmental Biology* 36, 8–23.

Johansson, J.A. and Headon, D.J. (2014) Regionalisation of the skin. *Seminars in Cell & Developmental Biology* 25–26, 3–10.

Jung, H.S., Francis-West, P.H., Widelitz, R.B., Jiang, T.X., Ting-Berreth, S. *et al.* (1998) Local inhibitory action of BMPs and their relationships with activators in feather formation: implications for periodic patterning. *Developmental Biology* 196, 11–23.

Kerje, S., Sharma, P., Gunnarsson, U., Kim, H., Bagchi, S. *et al.* (2004) The Dominant white, Dun and Smoky color variants in chicken are associated with insertion/deletion polymorphisms in the *PMEL17* gene. *Genetics* 168, 1507–1518.

Lamichhaney, S., Berglund, J., Almen, M.S., Maqbool, K., Grabherr, M. *et al.* (2015) Evolution of Darwin's finches and their beaks revealed by genome sequencing. *Nature* 518, 371–375.

Le Douarin, N.M., Creuzet, S., Couly, G. and Dupin, E. (2004) Neural crest cell plasticity and its limits. *Development* 131, 4637–4650.

Ludwig, A.W. and Boas, N.F. (1950) The effects of testosterone on the connective tissue of the comb of the cockerel. *Endocrinology* 46, 291–298.

Mattey, D.L. and Garrod, D.R. (1985) Mutual desmosome formation between all binary combinations of human, bovine, canine, avian and amphibian cells: desmosome formation is not tissue- or species-specific. *Journal of Cell Science* 75, 377–399.

Merat, P. (1986) Potential usefulness of the Na (naked neck) gene in poultry production. *World's Poultry Science Journal* 42, 124–142.

Mou, C., Pitel, F., Gourichon, D., Vignoles, F., Tzika, A. *et al.* (2011) Cryptic patterning of avian skin confers a developmental facility for loss of neck feathering. *PLOS Biology* 9, e1001028.

Noramly, S. and Morgan, B.A. (1998) BMPs mediate lateral inhibition at successive stages in feather tract development. *Development* 125, 3775–3787.

Ortolani-Machado, C., De Freitas, P., Borges, M.E. and Faraco, C. (2008) Special features of dermal melanocytes in white silky chicken embryos. *Anatomical Record* 291, 55–64.

Oster, G.F., Murray, J.D. and Harris, A.K. (1983) Mechanical aspects of mesenchymal morphogenesis. *Journal of Embryology and Experimental Morphology* 78, 83–125.

Painter, K.J., Hunt, G.S., Wells, K.L., Johansson, J.A. and Headon, D. J. (2012) Towards an integrated experimental-theoretical approach for assessing the mechanistic basis of hair and feather morphogenesis. *Interface Focus* 2, 433–450.

Parakkal, P.F. and Matoltsy, A.G. (1968) An electron microscopic study of developing chick skin. *Journal of Ultrastructure Research* 23, 403–416.

Pass, D.A. (1995) Normal anatomy of the avian skin and feathers. *Seminars in Avian and Exotic Pet Medicine* 4, 152–160.

Perez-Torres, A. and Ustarroz-Cano, M. (2001) Demonstration of Birbeck (Langerhans cells) granules in the normal chicken epidermis. *Journal of Anatomy* 199, 493–497.

Pick, L. (2016) Hox genes, evo-devo, and the case of the *ftz* gene. *Chromosoma* 125, 535–551.

Pitel, F., Berge, R., Coquerelle, G., Crooijmans, R.P.M.A., Groenen, M.A.M. *et al.* (2000) Mapping the Naked Neck (NA) and Polydactyly (PO) mutants of the chicken with microsatellite molecular markers. *Genetics, Selection, Evolution* 32, 73–86.

Richardson, R.J., Hammond, N.L., Coulombe, P.A., Saloranta, C., Nousiainen, H.O. *et al.* (2014) Periderm prevents pathological epithelial adhesions during embryogenesis. *Journal of Clinical Investigation* 124, 3891–3900.

Saathoff, M., Blum, B., Quast, T., Kirfel, G. and Herzog, V. (2004) Simultaneous cell death and desquamation of the embryonic diffusion barrier during epidermal development. *Experimental Cell Research* 299, 415–426.

Sawyer, R.H. and Knapp, L.W. (2003) Avian skin development and the evolutionary origin of feathers. *Journal of Experimental Zoology. Part B, Molecular and Developmental Evolution* 298, 57–72.

Sengel, P. and Abbott, U.K. (1963) In vitro studies with scaleless mutant – interactions during feather and scale differentiation. *Journal of Heredity* 54, 255–262.

Shapiro, M.D., Kronenberg, Z., Li, C., Domyan, E.T., Pan, H. *et al.* (2013) Genomic diversity and evolution of the head crest in the rock pigeon. *Science* 339, 1063–1067.

Shinomiya, A., Kayashima, Y., Kinoshita, K., Mizutani, M., Namikawa, T. *et al.* (2012) Gene duplication of endothelin 3 is closely correlated with the hyperpigmentation of the internal organs (Fibromelanosis) in silky chickens. *Genetics* 190, 627–638.

Shyer, A.E., Rodrigues, A.R., Schroeder, G.G., Kassianidou, E., Kumar, S. *et al.* (2017) Emergent cellular self-organization and mechanosensation initiate follicle pattern in the avian skin. *Science* 357, 811–815.

Singh, C., Kumar, D. and Singh, Y. (2001) Potential usefulness of the plumage reducing naked neck (Na) gene in poultry production at normal and high ambient temperatures. *World's Poultry Science Journal* 57, 127–156.

Somes, R.G. (1992) Identifying the ptilopody (feathered shank) loci of the chicken. *Journal of Heredity* 83, 230–234.

Stettenheim, P.R. (2000) The integumentary morphology of modern birds – an overview. *American Zoologist* 40, 461–477.

Sun, Y.F., Liu, R.R., Zhao, G.P., Zheng, M.Q., Sun, Y. *et al.* (2015) Genome-wide linkage analysis identifies loci for physical appearance traits in chickens. *G3-Genes Genomes Genetics* 5, 2037–2041.

Thoma, F. (1999) Light and dark in chromatin repair: repair of UV-induced DNA lesions by photolyase and nucleotide excision repair. *EMBO Journal* 18, 6585–6598.

Thomas, A.J. and Erickson, C.A. (2008) The making of a melanocyte: the specification of melanoblasts from the neural crest. *Pigment Cell & Melanoma Research* 21, 598–610.

Ting-Berreth, S.A. and Chuong, C.M. (1996) Local delivery of TGF beta2 can substitute for placode epithelium to induce mesenchymal condensation during skin appendage morphogenesis. *Developmental Biology* 179, 347–359.

Vestergaard, K.S., Damm, B.I., Abbott, U.K. and Bildso, E.M. (1999) Regulation of dustbathing in feathered and featherless domestic chicks: the Lorenzian model revisited. *Animal Behaviour* 58, 1017–1025.

Vickrey, A.I., Domyan, E.T., Horvath, M.P. and Shapiro, M.D. (2015) Convergent evolution of head crests in two domesticated Columbids is associated with different missense mutations in EphB2. *Molecular Biology and Evolution* 32, 2657–2664.

Wang, Y., Gao, Y., Imsland, F., Gu, X., Feng, C. *et al.* (2012) The crest phenotype in chicken is associated with ectopic expression of HOXC8 in cranial skin. *PLOS ONE* 7, e34012.

Wells, K.L., Hadad, Y., Ben-Avraham, D., Hillel, J., Cahaner, A. *et al.* (2012) Genome-wide SNP scan of pooled DNA reveals nonsense mutation in FGF20 in the scaleless line of featherless chickens. *BMC Genomics* 13, 257.

Wetmore, A. (1936) The number of contour feathers in Passeriform and related birds. *The Auk* 53, 159–169.

Widelitz, R.B., Jiang, T.X., Noveen, A., Chen, C.W. and Chuong, C.M. (1996) FGF induces new feather buds from developing avian skin. *Journal of Investigative Dermatology* 107, 797–803.

Widelitz, R.B., Jiang, T.X., Lu, J. and Chuong, C.M. (2000) Beta-catenin in epithelial morphogenesis: conversion of part of avian foot scales into feather buds with a mutated beta-catenin. *Developmental Biology* 219, 98–114.

Wright, D., Boije, H., Meadows, J. R., Bed'hom, B., Gourichon, D. *et al.* (2009) Copy number variation in intron 1 of SOX5 causes the Pea-comb phenotype in chickens. *PLOS Genetics* 5, e1000512.

Wu, P., Jiang, T.X., Suksaweang, S., Widelitz, R.B. and Chuong, C.M. (2004) Molecular shaping of the beak. *Science* 305, 1465–1466.

Wu, W., Xu, R.F., Gu, X., Li, C.H. and Wu, C.X. (2008) Characterization of embryonic feather follicle development in the Chinese indigenous Jilin White goose. *Asian-Australasian Journal of Animal Sciences* 21, 346–352.

Yalcin, S., Testik, A., Ozkan, S., Settar, P., Celen, F. *et al.* (1997) Performance of naked neck and normal broilers in hot, warm, and temperate climates. *Poultry Science* 76, 930–937.

Yu, M., Yue, Z., Wu, P., Wu, D.Y., Mayer, J.A. *et al.* (2004) The developmental biology of feather follicles. *International Journal of Developmental Biology* 48, 181–191.

Zou, H.Y. and Niswander, L. (1996) Requirement for BMP signaling in interdigital apoptosis and scale formation. *Science* 272, 738–741.

PART II

Health and Welfare

CHAPTER 3
Feather Pecking in Laying Hens: Why They Do It, and Welfare Implications

Christine J. Nicol*

Royal Veterinary College, London, UK

ABSTRACT

Severe feather pecking in laying hens is a significant welfare problem, causing pain, increased susceptibility to infection and an increased risk of premature death. Severe feather pecking is strongly related to absent, inadequate or insufficient foraging opportunities or to dietary deficiencies. Management practices that acknowledge the importance of foraging and dietary factors have been shown to be protective against feather pecking in commercial flocks. Further progress in prevention and control will depend on a greater understanding of the causal basis of feather pecking, and differences in individual bird propensity to peck.

DIFFERENT FORMS OF FEATHER PECKING

There is more than one form of feather pecking. Early studies did not differentiate between these different forms but Savory (1995) observed that feather pecking could occur in a severe manner or in a gentle manner. Since that time researchers have been increasingly careful to distinguish between these forms. Gentle (GFP) and severe feather pecking (SFP) are not only visibly different in appearance, but they also seem to be influenced by different causal factors (Rodenburg *et al.*, 2013). Certainly, the consequences for hen welfare are very different, with only minor plumage damage associated with GFP. In contrast, pecking, pulling and removal of feathers during SFP causes pain for the recipient and is associated with increased feather loss and skin damage (Bilcik and Keeling, 1999; Pötszch *et al.*, 2001; Drake *et al.*, 2010; Lambton *et al.*, 2010), increased susceptibility to infection (Green *et al.*, 2000), reduced production (Nicol *et al.*,

*cnicol@rvc.ac.uk

2013), increased demand for food (Tauson and Svensson, 1980; Blokhuis and van der Haar, 1992) and increased rates of premature death (Yngvesson *et al.*, 2004; Nicol *et al.*, 2013; Rodenburg *et al.*, 2013). For these reasons, SFP is one of the greatest welfare (and sustainability) concerns in commercial laying hen production and it can be very difficult to prevent or control. SFP has been recorded during the rearing period (Lambton *et al.*, 2010; Gilani *et al.*, 2013) but the risk of this behaviour increases greatly as hens reach sexual maturity (Newberry *et al.*, 2007; Nicol *et al.*, 2013). Cloutier *et al.* (2000) observed a positive correlation between the frequency of SFP and frequency of cannibalistic behaviour in small laboratory-held groups of laying hens. SFP has also been associated with the onset of vent pecking (Lambton *et al.*, 2015), although both vent pecking and other forms of cannibalistic tissue pecking can arise spontaneously in the absence of prior feather pecking. It is important to note that not all birds within a flock will exhibit feather pecking and that the highest levels of damage can be inflicted by a very small proportion of pecking birds (Wechsler *et al.*, 1998; Daigle *et al.*, 2015; Piepho *et al.*, 2017).

Gentle feather pecking occurs commonly during both the rearing and laying periods (Lambton *et al.*, 2010; Gilani *et al.*, 2013; Nicol *et al.*, 2013). Some researchers have noted that GFP in young chicks can be directed primarily towards unfamiliar companions, perhaps as a method of establishing social familiarity (Riedstra and Groothuis, 2002), but GFP can also occur in a seemingly repetitive form directed towards familiar birds. Newberry *et al.* (2007) found correlations between GFP and SFP in laboratory studies, but in commercial flocks most researchers have not found a clear relationship between GFP and SFP (Rodenburg *et al.*, 2013). Indeed, in some studies, high levels of GFP have occurred alongside low levels of SFP (Hartcher *et al.*, 2015a)

Birds that have been deliberately selected for high or low tendency to feather peck provide a useful resource for understanding the links between feather pecking and other behaviours. A wealth of studies on such selected lines have shown that strains with a high feather pecking tendency also show greater stress responses (Kjaer and Guemene, 2009; Kjaer and Jorgensen, 2011), aggression (Bennewitz *et al.*, 2014; Grams *et al.*, 2015) fearfulness (Rodenburg *et al.*, 2010) locomotor activity (Kjaer, 2009; de Haas *et al.*, 2010; Kjaer *et al.*, 2015) and foraging behaviour (de Haas *et al.*, 2010). Birds selected for high feather pecking also show altered patterns of serotonin release and dopamine receptor type (Flisikowski *et al.*, 2009; Kops *et al.* 2014). Other studies examining individual variation within strains have sometimes (de Haas *et al.*, 2014a, b) but not always (Albentosa *et al.*, 2003; Hartcher *et al.*, 2015b) found associations between feather pecking and fearfulness. Often such an association may arise because birds that are pecked by others will become more fearful. However, there is also the possibility that fearful birds are more likely to initiate feather pecking. There is other evidence that negative early life experiences may predispose birds to become either feather peckers or victims. Negative events during early development have been found to reduce symmetry in a wide variety of species (Tuyttens, 2003), with studies on hens more specifically finding that feather peckers and victims have reduced bodily symmetry compared with controls (Tahamtani *et al.*, 2017).

AN OVERVIEW OF EVIDENCE

Early studies of feather pecking were mostly laboratory based and few in number, but between 1990 and 2010 the number of studies increased greatly, with an increasing trend towards studies conducted on commercial farms. Since 2010 the number of scientific studies on this topic has declined slightly, though the problem of feather pecking is far from resolved. With many hundreds of scientific studies available it would be useful to perform a statistical meta-analysis to obtain an overview of the most important risk factors and the most effective preventive measures. However, even a cursory analysis of the literature on feather pecking shows that this is not possible because of the diversity of investigations, approaches, experimental treatments and preventive measures that have been applied. To take just one example, studies of the effect of illumination level have used different light intensities, different light sources, or have examined the effects of applying light treatments at different ages, or the effects of gradually increasing or decreasing illumination level at the start or end of the day. The number of studies that are sufficiently similar to allow pooling of data or statistical results becomes vanishingly small. It is therefore possible only to conduct a qualitative review of the evidence and to try to reach a conclusion as to why hens engage in feather pecking.

WHY DO HENS PECK FEATHERS? INFLUENCE OF FORAGING AND DIETARY FACTORS

The predominant scientific view is that severe feather pecking is a form of redirected (but otherwise normal) ground-pecking or foraging motivation, rather than a form of aggression. Confined chickens generally spend less time ground-pecking and foraging than their free-living domesticated or wild-type ancestral counterparts, who spend up to 60% of daylight hours engaged in natural foraging activities. Given the opportunity, modern strains of laying hens will spend up to 50% of their daylight hours similarly engaged in foraging. The hypothesis that relates feather pecking to foraging activity was supported by early observations of an inverse relationship between these two behaviours (Blokhuis, 1986; Lindberg and Nicol, 1994; Aerni *et al.*, 2000). Klein *et al.* (2000) found differences between strains, not in the total time spent foraging in an enriched environment, but in the elements of foraging shown. Subsequent restriction of litter resulted in a decrease in foraging and an increase in object pecking in both strains, with one of the strains showing a more pronounced decrease in foraging-related scratching and a greater increase in feather pecking than the other.

A wealth of more recent studies have provided further supportive evidence for this general theory, by showing that factors that increase normal foraging behaviour are protective against feather pecking. Feeding mash rather than pellets has been strongly associated with a reduced risk of SFP and vent pecking on commercial farms (Green *et al.*, 2000; Lambton *et al.*, 2010). This is also an important risk factor for vent pecking, with Lambton *et al.* (2015) concluding that the risk was increased more than fivefold if flocks were fed pelleted feed compared with mash. Experimental trials have not always replicated this effect (Wahlstrom *et al.*, 2001) but generally, hens spend far more time foraging in diets presented in mash form, this in itself reducing the opportunity for feather pecking. Increased availability and quality of foraging substrate can greatly increase foraging time, resulting in birds that have less time and that are less motivated to peck each other's plumage (Klein *et al.*, 2000; Nicol *et al.*, 2001). Experimentally, it has been shown that the presence of a good-quality foraging substrate during the rearing period reduces feather pecking in young birds (Huber-Eicher and Sebö, 2001; Chow and Hogan, 2005; Gilani *et al.*, 2013). In a study of 47 rearing flocks, de Haas *et al.* (2014a) found that disruption or limitation of litter during the first 4 weeks of age increased SFP at 5 weeks of age and feather damage throughout the rearing period. Some authors have reported that the protective effect of early litter access can persist to adulthood (Nicol *et al.*, 2001; De Jong *et al.*, 2013a). However, one recent study found that the provision of hay to adult birds housed in laboratory pens reduced GFP but not SFP (Daigle *et al.*, 2014). The provision of foraging materials for older pullets also significantly reduced feather pecking behaviour (Dixon and Duncan, 2010). Good quality, dry, friable foraging materials are also strongly protective during the laying period both for birds housed in furnished cages (Huneau-Salaün *et al.*, 2014) and for birds in non-cage systems (Nicol *et al.*, 2001; De Jong *et al.*, 2013a, b; de Haas *et al.*, 2014b). Hens will use a wide variety of materials for foraging, including peat, sand, straw and wood shavings (Weeks and Nicol, 2006), though there may be some strain differences in substrate foraging preferences (Klein *et al.*, 2000).

Foraging opportunities are greatly increased if non-cage flocks have access to an outdoor range. Indirectly, good range usage can also facilitate foraging in the indoor litter area, which will be less crowded when a high proportion of the flock is outside. Many authors have found that use of an outdoor range reduces SFP and improves plumage condition (Green *et al.*, 2000; Nicol *et al.*, 2003; Lambton *et al.*, 2010; Heerkens *et al.*, 2015; reviewed by Pettersson *et al.*, 2016). Heerkens *et al.* (2015) found better feather scores on the back and better overall plumage scores in nine aviary flocks with access to the outside compared with 38 flocks that had no outdoor access.

The generally low fibre content of commercial diets is increasingly recognized as another factor related to the hen's foraging motivation. Satiety is harder to achieve when birds eat a low-fibre diet and their motivation to continue to forage and peck is maintained for longer than when they have ingested high-fibre feeds. In growing pullets housed on slats, a quantitative relationship was observed between the proportion of insoluble non-starch polysaccharides (NSP) in the diet and feeding time. Pullets spent proportionately longer feeding as NSP levels increase and this resulted in a proportional decrease in feather pecking, comb pecking and wire pecking (Qaisrani *et al.*, 2013). Additional NSP can also stimulate gizzard development, reduce proventriculus content and increase reflux of bile acids, thus aiding the digestibility of starches (Hetland *et al.*, 2003; Van Krimpen *et al.*, 2009).This also means that, contrary to some expectations, improved weight gain can be achieved in growing pullets fed higher-fibre diets

(Panaite *et al.*, 2016). The importance of increasing dietary fibre to safeguard against SFP is now widely supported by scientific studies (Hetland *et al.*, 2003; Van Krimpen *et al.*, 2009; Steenfeldt *et al.*, 2007; Elwinger *et al.*, 2008; Kriegseis *et al.*, 2012; Qaisrani *et al.*, 2013; Rodenburg *et al.*, 2013). Pullets that were provided with increased fibre in their diets showed reduced mortality due to cannibalism in the early lay period (Hartini *et al.*, 2002) and improved gut function (Hetland *et al.*, 2003; Van Krimpen *et al.*, 2009). For example, the onset of feather damage was delayed by 10 weeks by feeding hens a low-energy, coarsely ground, high-fibre diet compared with a normal layer ration (Van Krimpen *et al.*, 2008). In another study, feeding a high oil-and-fibre diet to free-range hens lowered the occurrence of vent damage (Kalmendal and Wall, 2012). Fermented forage sources can provide additional dietary fibre and reduce SFP with no adverse effects on production (Johannson *et al.*, 2016). The protective effects of additional fibre can be particularly strong when other risk factors are present, such as when diets are fed in pelleted form (Aerni *et al.*, 2000; El-Lethey *et al.*, 2000). In free-range systems some hens have the opportunity to ingest green fibrous material. This is both a potential benefit (in increasing fibre levels) and a drawback if the overall diet becomes unbalanced. Despite this positive evidence about the protective effects of increased fibre, and its relatively low cost, most commercial rations are still formulated with relatively low fibre levels, due to practical and technical reasons, including dietary bulk, transport and storage costs, and issues concerning waste disposal.

If dietary fibre is lacking birds may turn towards other fibre sources, including wood shavings (Hetland and Svihus, 2007) and, pertinently in the context of this review, feathers from other birds (Harlander-Matauschek *et al.*, 2006; Harlander-Matauschek and Häusler, 2009). Birds that learn to obtain fibre by pulling out feathers from their companions (rather than simply ingesting feathers that have been naturally shed) may cause significant plumage damage within a flock. In one experiment, hens with poor group-level plumage scores were observed to direct more pecking towards single feathers placed on the pen floor, and were more likely to ingest these feathers, than hens with good group-level plumage scores (Hartcher *et al.*, 2016). Similarly, older hens with poorer plumage scores were also more likely to peck at and eat loose feathers placed on the pen floor (Hartcher *et al.*, 2016) and birds that had been deliberately selected for high levels of feather pecking were more likely to eat loose feathers than controls (Meyer *et al.*, 2013; Bőgelein *et al.*, 2015). Although the causal relationship between feather eating and feather pecking is not yet clear (Hartcher *et al.*, 2016) there are suggestions that birds are seeking additional fibre or other nutrients supplied by feathers. In laboratory experiments, the inclusion of 10% shredded feathers to the diet reduced SFP bouts and improved feather condition (Kriegseis *et al.*, 2012).

Inadequate amino acid and protein levels can also contribute to the initiation and continuance of feather pecking. Plant-based diets have been linked with more vigorous feather pecking than diets that included fish, meat or bone meal (McKeegan *et al.*, 2001; Van Krimpen *et al.*, 2011). The mechanisms underlying these effects are not fully understood. However, it is known that the amino acid content of a diet can have direct effects on neurotransmitters and behaviour. For example, the large amino acids tryptophan and tyrosine can pass through the blood–brain barrier and alter brain levels of serotonin and dopamine, respectively. A recent study found no relationship between plasma levels of large amino acids and feather pecking behaviour, though birds with relatively low levels of tryptophan showed a tendency to increased aggression (Birkl *et al.*, 2017). Much further work remains to be done to elucidate the role of amino acids on the brain biology and tendency to feather peck in chickens.

Changes in diet, particularly if the new diet is of lower nutritional quality or contains less preferred ingredients than the previous diet, are a strong risk factor for the development of injurious pecking (Green *et al.*, 2000; Dixon and Nicol, 2008). This is possibly because birds hesitate or are reluctant to feed on the new diet initially and their foraging motivation therefore remains high and unsatisfied, leading them to explore more harmful pecking options. Gilani *et al.* (2013) reported a substantial reduction in risk of feather pecking if the number of diet changes during the rearing period was reduced. Birds that have been deliberately selected for high feather pecking in scientific experiments also show signs of increased feeding (particularly hunting) motivation (De Haas *et al.*, 2010) and have differing expression of genes concerned with nutrient absorption and the regulation of glucose homeostasis (Brunberg *et al.*, 2011). In some cases, birds that initiate severe, cannibalistic tissue pecking appear to chase and hunt their companions as if they were prey.

MANAGEMENT PRACTICES TO PREVENT AND CONTROL FEATHER PECKING

Adult birds

Recognizing the importance of allowing birds to forage is a necessary foundation for designing management practices to prevent or reduce the spread of feather pecking. For example, non-cage flocks are often restricted to wire or slatted areas of the laying house for some days or weeks after transfer with the aim of encouraging birds to use the nest boxes for laying, but this means that young hens will be unable to access foraging materials. This also applies if young free-range hens are prevented from accessing the outdoor range for some weeks after transfer to the laying house. It would therefore be predicted that such temporary restriction would increase the risk of SFP.

Strong evidence that temporary exclusion from litter areas does increase SFP comes from observational studies on commercial farms (Nicol *et al.*, 2003; Lambton *et al.*, 2010) but a smaller-scale experimental study found contrary evidence that temporary restriction could actually improve plumage condition (Alm *et al.*, 2015). This may be because keeping newly transferred birds close to important resources such as food, water and nest boxes may have outweighed the negative effects of temporary litter restriction. Given uncertainties about costs and benefits of temporary restriction, a safer approach is to provide additional foraging materials on the slatted areas during the restriction phase or to allow young birds to access the litter floor area for short periods during the afternoons, once egg laying has largely been completed. Early access to the outdoor range has been shown to improve plumage condition (Petek *et al.*, 2015).

Additional measures can be taken to encourage harmless foraging and pecking behaviour in commercial flocks of hens. These include the provision of hay bales (Daigle *et al.*, 2014), pecking strings (Jones *et al.*, 2000; McAdie *et al.*, 2005), pecking objects (e.g. a wooden board with attached small stones: Moroki and Tanaka, 2016) and pecking blocks (in cages: Holcman *et al.*, 2008; or in non-cage flocks: Pettersson *et al.*, 2017). Such provision should be seen as an addition and not a substitute for a good litter substrate. Foraging materials were significantly more effective in reducing feather pecking than other enrichments such as dust-bathing substrates, or novel objects (Dixon *et al.*, 2010). Another study found a positive effect of environmental enrichment (pecking strings, whole oats and increased litter depth provided from 12 days of age) during the rearing period, but the effect did not persist or was not sufficiently strong to improve plumage condition when the birds were 43 weeks of age (Hartcher *et al.*, 2015a).

Other practices that alter the risk of SFP in non-cage flocks include higher light intensities during the laying period (Kjaer and Vestergaard, 1999; Drake *et al.*, 2010; Mohammed *et al.*, 2010), flock size and stocking density (Nicol *et al.*, 1999; Zimmerman *et al.*, 2006; Steenfeldt and Nielsen, 2015) and the general health status of the flock (Green *et al.*, 2000; Heerkens *et al.*, 2015). Practical and feasible management strategies that maintain bird health and permit high levels of foraging behaviour have been devised by a process of extensive scientific review and stakeholder engagement (Lambton *et al.*, 2013). Thorough and extensive tests of the efficacy of these management strategies in long-term trials of 100 commercial non-cage flocks in the UK were highly encouraging. The more strategies implemented on commercial farms, the lower was the risk of GFP, SFP and the better the plumage condition of the birds (Lambton *et al.*, 2013). Subsequent work has compared 14 commercial free-range farms in Year 1 (before management strategies introduced) and then in Year 2 (after management strategies introduced). The strategies in this study were ‘pecking pans’ containing a particulate pecking block, wind chimes that made a noise when pecked, and long, narrow shelters designed to bridge the gap between the hen house and the outer range areas and therefore encourage range use. The overall effect of these measures was to improve range use and decrease both GFP and SFP (Pettersson *et al.*, 2017).

Chicks and pullets

Domestic chicks are hatched commercially in large incubators and reared without a mother hen. In a natural situation, chicks would spend much of their time being brooded by the mother hen, resting close to her body in conditions of warmth and darkness. Chicks that have been raised by a mother hen show less SFP than non-brooded chicks and these effects can persist into adulthood (Shimmura *et al.*, 2015). An exciting new avenue of research is to consider whether aspects of maternal care can be simulated under commercial conditions.

Dark brooders provide heat under a canopy of dark fringes, simulating the presence and function of a mother hen to some extent. Dark brooders synchronize chick behaviour (Riber *et al.*, 2007) and can reduce feather pecking very substantially (Jensen *et al.*, 2006; Gilani *et al.*, 2012; Riber and Guzman, 2016, 2017). This is possibly because active chicks do not encounter and direct exploratory pecks at resting chicks, but direct their active pecking behaviour towards the floor substrate. Minor differences in space allowance and management of the dark brooders does not have any significant impact on their beneficial effects (Riber and Guzman, 2017). The introduction of dark brooders on commercial rearing farms has also been highly successful (Gilani *et al.*, 2012). Compared with controls, flocks reared with dark brooders performed significantly less SFP and had lower proportions of birds with missing feathers. The benefits of simulating other aspects of maternal care are now being investigated. It has been shown, for example, that playback of maternal calls can buffer stress responses in chicks (Edgar *et al.*, 2015) but the longer-term effects of such manipulations on adult feather pecking have not yet been studied.

During the rearing period, factors that have been shown to increase feather pecking include higher or more variable sound levels (Gilani *et al.*, 2013), which may interrupt resting behaviour, and a lack of perches (Gunnarsson *et al.*, 1999; Huber-Eicher and Audigé, 1999). Other risk factors relate to disruptions or limitations of foraging behaviour. For example, the use of bell drinkers and high stocking densities increase the risk of feather pecking possibly by increasing the risk of wet or poor-quality litter (Bestman *et al.*, 2009; Drake *et al.*, 2010). A high number of diet changes during the rearing period will increase the risk of birds showing neophobic responses to new diets and redirecting their pecking motivation to other birds and this may explain the strong association seen between diet change and feather pecking (Gilani *et al.*, 2013). Minimizing change in management practice, housing design and diet between the rearing and the laying periods (Drake *et al.*, 2010) or effecting an early transfer to allow hens time to acclimatize to laying houses before the onset of lay (Bestman and Wagenaar, 2003) may be beneficial in reducing the risk of feather pecking in the early laying period. Given known associations between fearfulness and feather pecking, it may also be beneficial to rear birds under conditions that reduce fearfulness in adult birds (e.g. Brantsaeter *et al.*, 2017), though this remains to be fully tested. Higher light intensities during the rearing period have not, however, been shown to increase the risk of SFP (Hartini *et al.*, 2002).

BEAK TRIMMING

Beak trimming is very often employed as a preventive practice with the aim of reducing SFP and of reducing skin damage and mortality should feather pecking occur. There is some evidence that the practice is partially effective in these aims, as beak-trimmed pullets perform less SFP than birds with intact beaks (Gilani *et al.*, 2013; Hartcher *et al.*, 2015a), and the plumage condition of beak-trimmed birds is generally better (Lambton *et al.*, 2013; Sepeur *et al.*, 2015) unless additional special measures are taken, as in some small, organic flocks. Beak trimming is also associated with slightly reduced mortality in non-cage flocks (Weeks *et al.*, 2016).

Despite the benefits, the practice of beak trimming is contested on ethical grounds because it causes pain, and it compromises bird perception and sensory function. Hot-blade trimming of young chicks or pullets causes both short-term and chronic pain and stress (reviewed in Janczak and Riber, 2015). For this reason, hot-blade trimming is being replaced in many countries by an infrared (IR) procedure conducted at the hatchery. Chicks are restrained by their heads and IR energy is directed towards the tip of the beak. The beak tip drops off some days after treatment with only limited re-growth, due to damage to the tissue germ layers. IR trimming is thought to cause less pain but this conclusion is tentative (Dennis *et al.*, 2009; Nicol *et al.*, 2013). Birds that have been IR trimmed still show behavioural changes in comparison with untrimmed controls, particularly reduced feed intake and activity in the weeks after the procedure (reviewed in Janczak and Riber, 2015). In the longer term, birds that have been beak trimmed are less able to remove ecto-parasites (Mullens *et al.*, 2010; Chen *et al.*, 2011; Vezzoli *et al.*, 2015) and their navigational ability is reduced (Freire *et al.*, 2011).

The question thus arises as to whether commercial flocks of birds can be kept with intact beaks without their welfare being reduced by SFP and associated injury and disease. This may be easier to achieve in furnished or enriched cage systems than in non-cage systems, where overall mortality levels for intact-beak birds can be very low (e.g. Janczak and Riber, 2015). However, the potential to add meaningful enrichment to cages is reduced compared with non-cage systems, and enrichments that have been trialled so far have reduced pecking behaviour but had less of an effect on plumage cover and mortality than expected (Morrissey *et al.*, 2016). The consequences of keeping non-cage flocks with intact beaks was assessed in a recent UK trial. No problems were detected during rear, but outcomes during the laying period were highly variable (Nicol, 2015). Farms that had previously kept intact-beak flocks showed a significant improvement in end-of-lay mortality and plumage condition when they implemented additional management strategies. However, farms that transitioned from beak-trimmed to intact-beak flocks had no improvement in mortality or plumage condition, despite implementing additional management strategies. In these flocks, the positive effects of the management strategies were countered by the increased risks of keeping intact-beak birds (Nicol, 2015). More generally, this study shows that improvements in the welfare of intact-beak flocks can be obtained with increased experience and attention to management, something also borne out by the experience of developing new non-cage housing systems in The Netherlands (Spoelstra *et al.*, 2013).

Overall, the scientific evidence suggests that management innovations that increase the time that pullets and hens spend in 'healthy' foraging activity, and that allow birds to rest and perch, can lead to significant and substantial reductions in feather pecking and improvements in plumage condition. However, these management practices will act in concert with genetic influences (reviewed elsewhere) to create a highly complex system. Studies that consider both genetic and environment effects under commercial conditions are still needed to resolve the ongoing problem of feather pecking in laying hens.

REFERENCES

Aerni, V., El-Lethey, H. and Wechsler, B. (2000) Effect of foraging material and food form on feather pecking in laying hens. *British Poultry Science* 41, 16–21.

Albentosa, M.J., Kjaer, J.B. and Nicol, C.J. (2003) Strain and age differences in behaviour, fear response and pecking tendency in laying hens. *British Poultry Science* 44, 333–344

Alm, M., Wall, H., Holm, L., Wichman, A., Palme, R. and Tauson, R. (2015) Welfare and performance in layers following temporary exclusion from the litter area on introduction to the later facility. *Poultry Science* 94, 565–573.

Bennewitz, J., Bogelein, S., Stratz, P., Rodehutscord, M., Piepho, H.P., Kjaer, J.B. and Bessei, W. (2014) Genetic parameters for feather pecking and aggressive behaviour in a large F2-cross of laying hens using generalized linear mixed models. *Poultry Science* 93, 810–817

Bestman, M.W.P. and Wagenaar, J.P. (2003) Farm level factors associated with feather pecking in organic laying hens. *Livestock Production Science* 80, 133–140

Bestman, M., Koene, P. and Wagenaar, J.-P. (2009) Influence of farm factors on the occurrence of feather pecking in organic reared hens and their predictability for feather pecking in the laying period. *Applied Animal Behaviour Science* 121, 120–124

Bilcik, B. and Keeling, L.J. (1999) Changes in feather condition in relation to feather pecking and aggressive behaviour in laying hens. *British Poultry Science* 40, 444–451

Birkl, P., Franke, L., Rodenburg, T.B., Ellen, E. and Harlander-Matauschek, A. (2017) A role for plasma aromatic amino acids in injurious pecking behaviour in laying hens. *Physiology and Behavior* 175, 88–96.

Blokhuis, H.J. (1986) Feather pecking in poultry – its relation with ground pecking. *Applied Animal Behaviour Science* 16, 63–67

Blokhuis, H.J. and van der Haar, J.W. (1992) Effects of pecking incentives during rearing on feather pecking of laying hens. *British Poultry Science* 33(1), 17–24. doi: 10.1080/00071669208417440

Bőgelein, S., Kjaer, J.B., Bennewitz, J. and Bessei, W. (2015) The phenotypic interrelationships between feather pecking, being feather pecked, feather eating, feather score, fear, body weight and egg production traits in a F2-cross of White Leghorn lines selected for high and low severe feather pecking. *European Poultry Science* 79. doi: 10.1399/eps.2015.84

Brantsaeter, M., Tahamtani, F.M., Nordgreen, J., Sandberg, E., Hansen, T.B. *et al.* (2017) Access to litter during rearing and environmental enrichment during production reduce fearfulness in adult laying hens. *Applied Animal Behaviour Science* 189, 49–56.

Brunberg, E., Jensen, P., Isaksson, A. and Keeling, L.J. (2011) Feather pecking behaviour in laying hens: hypothalamic gene expression in birds performing and receiving pecks. *Poultry Science* 90, 1145–1152

Chen, B.L., Haith, K.L. and Mullens, B.A. (2011) Beak condition drives abundance and grooming-mediated competitive asymmetry in a poultry ectoparasite community. *Parasitology* 138, 748–757.

Chow, A and Hogan, J.A. (2005) The development of feather pecking in Burmese red junglefowl: the influence of early experience with exploratory-rich environments. *Applied Animal Behaviour Science* 93, 283–294.

Cloutier S., Newberry, R.C., Forster, C.T. and Girsberger, K.M. (2000) Does pecking at inanimate stimuli predict cannibalistic behaviour in domestic fowl? *Applied Animal Behaviour Science* 66, 119–133.

Daigle, C.L., Rodenburg, T.B., Bolhuis, J.E., Swanson, J.C. and Siegford, J.M. (2014) Use of dynamic and rewarding environmental enrichment to alleviate feather pecking in non-cage laying hens. *Applied Animal Behaviour Science* 161, 75–85.

Daigle, C.L., Rodenburg, T.B., Bolhuis, J.E., Swanson, J.C. and Siegford, J.M. (2015) Individual consistency of feather pecking behaviour in laying hens: once a feather pecker always a feather pecking? *Frontiers in Veterinary Science* 2, 6. doi: 10.3389/fvets2015.00006

De Haas, E.N., Nielsen, B.L., Buitenhuis, A.J. and Rodenburg, T.B. (2010) Selection on feather pecking affects response to novelty and foraging behaviour in laying hens. *Applied Animal Behaviour Science* 124, 90–96.

De Haas, E.N., Bolhuis, J.E., Kemp, B., Groothuis, T.G.G., Rodenburg, T.B. (2014a) Parents and early life environment affect behavioural development of laying hen chickens. *PLOS ONE* e90577.

De Haas, E.N., Bolhuis, J.E., de Jong, I.C., Kemp, B., Janczac, A.M. and Rodenburg, T.B. (2014b) Predicting feather damage in laying hens during the laying period. Is it the past or is it the present? *Applied Animal Behaviour Science* 160, 75–85

De Jong, I.C., Reuvekamp, B.F.J. and Gunnink, H. (2013a) Can substrate in early rearing prevent feather pecking in adult laying hens? *Animal Welfare* 22, 305–314.

De Jong, I.C., Gunnink, H., Rommers, J.M. and Bracke, M.B.M. (2013b) Effect of substrate during early rearing on floor and feather pecking behaviour in young and adult laying hens. *Archiv fur Geflugelkunde* 77, 15–22.

Dennis, R.L., Fahey, A.G. and Cheng, H.W. (2009) Infrared beak treatment method compared with conventional hot-blade trimming in laying hens. *Poultry Science* 88, 38–43.

Dixon, G. and Nicol, C.J. (2008) The effect of diet change on the behaviour of layer pullets. *Animal Welfare* 17, 101–109.

Dixon, L.M. and Duncan, I.J.H. (2010) Changes in substrate access did not affect early feather-pecking behaviour in two strains of laying hen chicks. *Journal of Applied Animal Welfare Science* 13, 1–14.

Dixon, L.M., Duncan, I.J.H. and Mason, G.J. (2010) The effects of four types of enrichment on feather pecking behaviour in laying hens housed in barren environments. *Animal Welfare* 19, 429–435.

Drake, K.A., Donnelly, C.A. and Dawkins, M.S. (2010) Influence of rearing and lay risk factors on propensity for feather damage in laying hens. *British Poultry Science* 51, 725–733.

Edgar, J.E., Kelland, I., Held, S., Paul, E and Nicol, C.J. (2015) Effects of maternal vocalisations on the domestic chick stress response. *Applied Animal Behaviour Science* 171, 121–127.

El-Lethey, H., Aerni, V., Jungi, T.W. and Wechsler, B. (2000) Stress and feather pecking in laying hens in relation to housing conditions. *British Poultry Science* 41, 22–28.

Elwinger, K., Tufvesson, M., Lagekvist, G. and Tauson, R. (2008) Feeding layers of different genotypes in organic feed environments. *British Poultry Science* 49, 654–665.

Flisikowski, K., Schwarzenbacher, H., Wysocki, M., Weigend, S., Preisinger, R., Kjaer, J.B. and Fries, R. (2009) Variation in neighbouring genes of the dopaminergic and serotinergic systems affects feather pecking behaviour of laying hens. *Animal Genetics* 40, 192–199.

Freire, R., Eastwood, M.A. and Joyce, M. (2011) Minor beak trimming in chickens leads to loss of mechanoreception and magnetoreception. *Journal of Animal Science* 89, 1201–1206

Gilani, A.-M., Knowles, T.G. and Nicol, C.J. (2012) The effect of dark brooders on feather pecking on commercial farms. *Applied Animal Behaviour Science* 142, 42–50.

Gilani, A.-M., Knowles, T.G. and Nicol, C.J. (2013) The effect of rearing environment on feather pecking in young and adult laying hens. *Applied Animal Behaviour Science* 148, 54–63.

Grams, V., Bogelein,S., Grashorn, M.A., Bessei, W and Bennewitz, J. (2015) Quantitative genetic analysis of traits related to fear and feather pecking in laying hens. *Behavior Genetics* 45, 228–235.

Green, L.E., Lewis, K., Kimpton, A. and Nicol, C.J. (2000) Cross-sectional study of the prevalence of feather pecking in laying hens in alternative systems and its associations with management and disease. *Veterinary Record* 147, 233–238.

Gunnarsson, S., Keeling, L.J. and Svedburg, J. (1999) Effect of rearing factors on the prevalence of floor eggs, cloacal cannibalism and feather pecking in commercial flocks of loose housed laying hens. *British Poultry Science* 40, 12–18.

Harlander-Matauschek, A. and Häusler, K. (2009) Understanding feather eating behavior in laying hens. *Applied Animal Behaviour Science* 117, 35–41.
Harlander-Matauschek, A., Baes, C. and Bessei, W. (2006) The demand of laying hens for feathers and wood shavings. *Applied Animal Behaviour Science* 101, 102–110.
Hartcher, K.M., Tran, K.T.N., Wilkinson, S.J., Hemsworth, P.H., Thomson, P.C. and Cronin, G.M. (2015a) The effects of environmental enrichment and beak-trimming during the rearing period on subsequent feather damage due to feather-pecking in laying hens. *Poultry Science* 94, 852–859.
Hartcher, K.M., Tran, M.K.T.N., Wilkinson, S.J., Hemsworth, P.H., Thomson, P.C. and Cronin, G.M. (2015b) Plumage damage in free-range laying hens: behavioural characteristics in the rearing period and the effects of environmental enrichment and beak-trimming. *Applied Animal Behaviour Science* 164, 64–72.
Hartcher, K.M., Hemsworth, P.H., Wilkinson, S.J., Thomson, P.C. and Cronin, G.M. (2016) The association between plumage damage and feather-eating in free-range laying hens. *Animal* 10(5), 854–862.
Hartini, S., Choct, M., Hinch, G., Kocher, A. and Nolan, J.V. (2002) Effects of light intensity during rearing and beak trimming and dietary fiber sources on mortality, egg production and performance of ISA brown laying hens. *Journal of Applied Poultry Research* 11,104–110.
Heerkens, J.L.T., Delezie, E., Kempen, I., Zoons, J., Ampe, B., Rodenburg, T.B. and Tuyttens, F.A.M. (2015) Specific characteristics of the aviary housing system affect plumage condition, mortality and production in laying hens. *Poultry Science* 94(9), 2008–2017.
Hetland, H. and Svihus, B. (2007) Inclusion of dust bathing materials affects nutrient digestion and gut physiology of layers. *Journal of Applied Poultry Research* 16, 22–26.
Hetland, H., Svihus, B., Lervik, S. and Moe, R. (2003) Effect of feed structure on performance and welfare in laying hens housed in conventional and furnished cages. *Acta Agriculturae Scandinavica Section A – Animal Science* 53, 92–100.
Holcman, A., Gorjanc, G. and Stuhec, I. (2008) Porous concrete block as an environmental enrichment device increases activity of laying hens in cages. *Poultry Science* 87, 1714–1719.
Huber-Eicher, B. and Audigé, L. (1999) Analysis of risk factors for the occurrence of feather pecking in laying hen growers. *British Poultry Science* 40, 599–604.
Huber-Eicher, B. and Sebö, F. (2001) Reducing feather pecking when raising laying hen chicks in aviary systems. *Applied Animal Behaviour Science* 73, 59–68.
Huneau-Salaün, A., Guinebretière, M. and Michel, V. (2014) Effect of substrate provision on performance and behaviour of laying hens in the pecking and scratching area of furnished cages. *British Poultry Science* 55(4), 409–418.
Janczak, A.M. and Riber, A.B. (2015) Review of rearing-related factors affecting the welfare of laying hens. *Poultry Science* 94, 1454–1469
Jensen, A.B., Palme, R and Forkman, B. (2006) Effect of brooders on feather pecking and cannibalism in domestic fowl (*Gallus gallus domesticus*). *Applied Animal Behaviour Science* 99, 287–300.
Johannson, S.G., Raginski, C., Schwean-Lardner, K. and Classen, H.L. (2016) Providing laying hens in group-housed enriched cages with access to barley silage reduces aggressive and feather pecking behaviour. *Canadian Journal of Animal Science* 96, 161–171.
Jones, R.B., Carmichael, N.L. and Rayner, E. (2000) Pecking preferences and pre-dispositions in domestic chicks: implications for the development of environmental enrichment devices. *Applied Animal Behaviour Science* 69, 291–312
Kalmendal, R. and Wall, H. (2012) Effects of a high oil and fibre diet and supplementary roughage on performance, injurious pecking and foraging activities in two layer hybrids. *British Poultry Science* 53, 153–161.

Kjaer, J.B. (2009) Feather pecking in domestic fowl is genetically related to locomotor activity levels: implications for a hyperactivity disorder model of feather pecking. *Behavior Genetics* 39, 564–570.

Kjaer, J.B. and Guemene, D. (2009) Adrenal reactivity in lines of domestic fowl selected on feather pecking behaviour. *Physiology and Behavior* 96, 370–373.

Kjaer, J.B. and Jorgensen, H. (2011) Heart rate variability in domestic chicken lines genetically selected on feather pecking behaviour. *Genes Brain and Behavior* 10, 747–755.

Kjaer, J.B. and Vestergaard, K.S. (1999) Development of feather pecking in relation to light intensity. *Applied Animal Behaviour Science* 62, 243–254.

Kjaer, J.B., Wuerbel, H. and Schrader, L. (2015) Perseveration in a guessing task by laying hens selected for high or low levels of feather pecking does not support classification of feather pecking as a stereotypy. *Applied Animal Behaviour Science* 168, 56–60.

Klein, T., Zeltner, E. and Huber-Eicher, B. (2000) Are genetic differences in foraging behaviour of laying hen chicks paralleled by hybrid-specific differences in feather pecking? *Applied Animal Behaviour Science* 70, 143–155.

Kops, M.S., Kjaer, J.B., Gunturkun, O., Westphal, K.G.C., Korte-Bouws, G.A.H. *et al.* (2014) Serotonin release in the caudal nidopallium of adult laying hens genetically selected for high and low feather pecking behavior: an in vivo microdialysis study. *Behavioural Brain Research* 268, 81–87.

Kriegseis, I., Bessei, W., Meyer, B. Zentek, J., Wuerbel, H. and Harlander-Matauschek, A. (2012) Feather pecking responses of laying hens to feather and cellulose-based rations fed during rearing. *Poultry Science* 91, 1514–1521.

Lambton, S.L., Knowles, T.G., Yorke, C. and Nicol, C.J. (2010) The risk factors affecting the development of gentle and severe feather pecking in loose housed laying hens. *Applied Animal Behaviour Science* 123, 32–42.

Lambton, S.L., Nicol, C.J., Friel, M., Main, D.C.J., McKinstry, J.L. *et al.* (2013) A bespoke management package can reduce the levels of injurious pecking in loose housed laying hen flocks. *Veterinary Record* 172, 423–430.

Lambton, S.L., Knowles, T.G., Yorke, C. and Nicol, C.J. (2015) The risk factors affecting the development of vent pecking and cannibalism in free-range and organic laying hens. *Animal Welfare* 24, 101–111.

Lindberg, A.C. and Nicol, C.J. (1994) An evaluation of the effect of operant feeders on welfare of hens maintained on litter. *Applied Animal Behaviour Science* 41, 211–227.

McAdie, T.M., Keeling, L.J., Blokhuis, H.J. and Jones, R.B. (2005) Reduction in feather pecking and improvement of feather condition with the presentation of a string device to chickens. *Applied Animal Behaviour Science* 93, 67–80.

McKeegan, D.E.F., Savory, C.J., MacLeod, M.G. and Mitchell, M.A. (2001) Development of pecking damage in layer pullets in relation to dietary protein source. *British Poultry Science* 42, 33–42

Meyer, B., Zentek, J. and Harlander-Matauschek, A. (2013) Differences in intestinal microbial metabolites in laying hens with high and low levels of repetitive feather-pecking behaviour. *Physiology and Behavior* 110, 96–101

Mohammed, H.H., Grashorn, M.A. and Bessei, W. (2010) The effects of lighting conditions on the behaviour of laying hens. *Archiv fur Geflugelkunde* 74, 197–202.

Moroki, Y. and Tanaka, T. (2016) A pecking device as an environmental enrichment for caged laying hens. *Animal Science Journal* 87, 1055–1062.

Morrissey, K.L.H., Brocklehurst, S., Baker, L., Widowski, T.M. and Sandilands, V. (2016) Can non-beak treated hens be kept in commercial furnished cages? Exploring the effects of strain and extra environmental enrichment on behaviour, feather cover and mortality. *Animals* 6(3), 17. doi: 10.3390/ani6030017

Mullens, B.A., Chen, B.L. and Owen, J.P. (2010) Beak condition and cage density determine abundance and spatial distribution of northern fowl mites, *Ornithonyssus sylviarum*, and chicken body lice, *Menacanthus stramineus*, on caged laying hens. *Poultry Science* 89, 2565–2572.

Newberry, R.C., Keeling, L.J., Estevez, I. and Bilcik, B. (2007) Behaviour when young as a predictor of severe feather pecking in adult laying hens: the redirected foraging hypothesis revisited. *Applied Animal Behaviour Science* 107, 262–274.

Nicol, C.J. (2015) A study to test the effectiveness of management strategies in reducing injurious pecking of laying hens with intact beaks in non cage systems. Defra Final Report. Department for Environment, Food & Rural Affairs, London. Available at: sciencesearch.defra.gov.uk/Document.aspx?Document=13041_AW1145Finalreport.pdf (accessed 4 October 2018).

Nicol, C.J., Gregory, N.G., Knowles, T.G., Parkman, I.D. and Wilkins, L.J. (1999) Differential effects of increased stocking density, mediated by increased flock size, on feather pecking and aggression in laying hens. *Applied Animal Behaviour Science* 65, 137–152

Nicol, C.J., Lindberg, A.C., Phillips, A.J., Pope, S.J., Wilkins, L.J. and Green, L.E. (2001) Influences of prior exposure to wood shavings on feather pecking, dustbathing and foraging in adult laying hens. *Applied Animal Behaviour Science* 73, 141–155.

Nicol, C.J., Pötszch, C., Lewis, K. and Green, L.E. (2003) Matched concurrent case-control study of risk factors for feather pecking in hens on free-range commercial farms in the UK. *British Poultry Science* 44, 515–523.

Nicol, C.J., Bestman, M., Gilani, A.M., De Haas, E.N., De Jong, I.C., Lambton, S. *et al.* (2013) The prevention and control of feather pecking: application to commercial systems. *World's Poultry Science Journal* 69, 775–788.

Panaite, C.V., Criste, R.D., Dragotoiu, D., Panaite, T.D. and Olteanu, M. (2016) Effect of crude fibre concentration in pullet diets (9–16 weeks) on their subsequent performance. *Agrolife Scientific Journal* 5, 161–167.

Petek, M., Topal, E. and Cavusoglu, E. (2015) Effects of age at first access to range area on pecking behaviour and plumage quality of free-range layer chickens. *Archiv for Tierzucht* 58, 85–91.

Pettersson, I.C., Freire, R. and Nicol, C.J. (2016) Factors affecting ranging behaviour in commercial free-range hens. *World's Poultry Science Journal* 72, 137–149.

Pettersson, I.C., Weeks, C.A. and Nicol, C.J. (2017) Provision of a resource package reduces feather pecking and improves ranging distribution on free-range layer farms. *Applied Animal Behaviour Science* 195, 60–66.

Piepho, H.-P., Lutz, V., Kjaer, J.B., Grashorn, M., Bennewitz, J. and Bessei, W. (2017) The presence of extreme feather peckers in groups of laying hens. *Animal* 11, 500–506.

Pötzsch, C.J., Lewis, K., Nicol, C.J. and Green, L.E. (2001) A cross-sectional study of the prevalence of vent pecking in laying hens in alternative systems and its associations with feather pecking, management and disease. *Applied Animal Behaviour Science* 74, 259–272.

Qaisrani, S.N., van Krimpen, M.M. and Kwakkel, R.P. (2013) Effects of dietary dilution source and dilution level on feather damage, performance, behaviour and litter condition in pullets. *Poultry Science* 92, 591–602.

Riber, A.B. and Guzman, D.A. (2016) Effects of dark brooders on behaviour and fearfulness in layers. *Animals* 6(1), 3. doi: 10.3390/ani6010003.

Riber, A.B. and Guzman, D.A. (2017) Effects of different types of dark brooders on injurious pecking damage and production-related traits at rear and lay in layers. *Poultry Science* 96, 3529–3538

Riber, A.B., Nielsen, B.L., Ritz, C. and Forkman, B. (2007) Diurnal activity cycles and synchrony in layer hen chicks (*Gallus gallus domesticus*). *Applied Animal Behaviour Science* 108, 276–287.

Riedstra, B. and Groothuis, T.G.G. (2002) Early feather pecking as a form of social exploration: the effect of group stability on feather pecking and tonic immobility in domestic chicks. *Applied Animal Behaviour Science* 77, 127–138.

Rodenburg, T.B., De Haas, E.N., Nielsen, B.L. and Buitenhuis, A.J. (2010) Fearfulness and feather damage in laying hens divergently selected for high and low feather pecking. *Applied Animal Behaviour Science* 128, 91–96.

Rodenburg, T.B., Van Krimpen, M.M., De Jong, I.C., De Haas, E.N., Kops, M.S. *et al.* (2013) The prevention and control of feather pecking in laying hens: identifying the underlying principles. *World's Poultry Science Journal* 69, 361–373.

Savory C.J. (1995) Feather pecking and cannibalism. *World's Poultry Science Journal* 51, 215–219.

Sepeur, S., Spindler, B., Schulze-Bisping, M., Habig, C., Andersson, R., Beverbach, M. and Kemper, N. (2015) Comparison of plumage condition of laying hens with intact and trimmed beaks kept on commercial farms. *European Poultry Science* 79. doi: 10.1399/eps.2015.116

Shimmura, T., Maruyama, Y., Fujino, S., Kamimura, E., Uetake, K. and Tanaka, T. (2015) Persistent effect of broody hens on behaviour of chickens. *Animal Science Journal* 86, 214–220.

Spoelstra, S.F., Koerkamp, P.W.G.G., Bos, A.P., Elzen, B. and Leenstra, F.R. (2013) Innovation for sustainable egg production: realigning production with societal demands in The Netherlands. *World's Poultry Science Journal* 69, 279–297.

Steenfeldt, S. and Nielsen, B.L. (2015) Welfare of organic laying hens kept at different indoor stocking densities in a multi-tier aviary system II: live weight, health measures and perching. *Animal* 9, 1518–1528.

Steenfeldt, S., Kjaer, J.B. and Engberg, R.M. (2007) Effect of feeding silages or carrots as supplements to laying hens on production performance, nutrient digestibility, gut structure, gut microflora and feather pecking behaviour. *British Poultry Science* 48, 454–468.

Tahamtani, F.M., Forkman, B., Hinrichsen, L.K. and Riber, A.B. (2017) Both feather peckers and victims are more asymmetrical than control hens. *Applied Animal Behaviour Science* 195, 67–71.

Tauson, R., and Svensson, S.A. (1980) Influence of plumage condition on the hens feed requirement. *Swedish Journal of Agricultural Research* 10(1), 35–39.

Tuyttens, F.A.M. (2003) Measures of developmental instability as integrated, a posterior indicators of farm animal welfare: a review. *Animal Welfare* 12, 535–540.

Van Krimpen, M.M., Kwakkel, R.P., van der Peet-Schwering, C.M.C., den Hartog, L.A. and Verstegen, M.W.A. (2008) Low dietary energy concentration, high nonstarch polysaccharide concentration, and coarse particle sizes of nonstarch polysaccharides affect the behaviour of feather-pecking prone laying hens. *Poultry Science* 87, 485–496.

Van Krimpen, M.M., Kwakkel, R.P., van der Peet-Schwering, C.M.C., den Hartog, L.A. and Verstegen, M.W.A. (2009) Effect of nutrient dilution and nonstarch polysaccharide concentration in rearing and laying diets on eating behaviour and feather damage of rearing and laying hens. *Poultry Science* 88, 759–773.

Van Krimpen, M.M., Kwakkel, R.P., van der Peet-Schwering, C.M.C., den Hartog, L.A. and Verstegen, M.W.A. (2011) Effects of dietary energy concentration, nonstarch polysaccharide concentration, and particle sizes of nonstarch polysaccharides on digesta mean retention time and gut development in laying hens. *British Poultry Science* 52, 730–741.

Vezzoli, G., Mullens, B. and Mench, J.A. (2015) Relationships between beak condition, preening behaviour and ectoparasite infestation levels in laying hens. *Poultry Science* 94, 1997–2007.

Wahlstrom, A., Tauson, R. and Elwinger, K. (2001) Plumage condition and health of aviary-kept hens fed mash or crumbled pellets. *Poultry Science* 80, 266–271.

Wechsler, B., Huber-Eicher, B. and Nash, D.R. (1998) Feather pecking in growers. A study with individually marked birds. *British Poultry Science* 39, 178–185.

Weeks, C.A. and Nicol, C.J. (2006) Behavioural needs, priorities and preferences of laying hens. *World's Poultry Science Journal* 62, 296–307.
Weeks, C.A., Lambton, S.L. and Williams, A.G. (2016) Implications for welfare, productivity and sustainability of the variation in reported levels of mortality for laying hen flocks kept in different housing systems: a meta-analysis of ten studies. *PLOS ONE* 11(1) e0146394.
Yngvesson, J., Keeling, L.J. and Newberry, R.C. (2004) Individual production differences do not explain cannibalistic behaviour in laying hens. *British Poultry Science* 45(4), 453–462.
Zimmerman, P.H, Lindberg, A.C., Pope, S.J., Glenm E., Bolhuis, J.E. and Nicol, C.J. (2006) The effect of stocking density, flock size and modified management on laying hen behaviour and welfare in a non-cage system. *Applied Animal Behaviour Science* 101, 111–124.

CHAPTER 4
Genetic Solutions to Reduce Injurious Pecking in Laying Hens

Esther D. Ellen* and Piter Bijma

Animal Breeding and Genomics, Wageningen University & Research, Wageningen, The Netherlands

ABSTRACT

Survival of commercial laying hens is an important trait. Feather pecking has a large effect on the survival of birds. To improve survival it is important to use quantitative genetic methods that take into account both the direct genetic effect (victim effect) and the indirect genetic effect (actor effect). For survival time, we found that the victim effect contributes 13–64% of total heritable variation, while the actor effect contributes 36–87% of total heritable variation. Together, they explain 15–26% of total phenotypic variation in survival time. Here we compare different breeding programme designs to identify the optimum selection strategy against mortality due to feather pecking. Results show that mortality due to feather pecking can be reduced using genetic approaches, taking into account direct and indirect genetic effects. We performed a selection experiment using selection based on relatives. Using this method enables selection against mortality due to feather pecking in laying hens. However, selection intensities were small. Genomic selection can be a promising tool to select against mortality due to feather pecking. Model predictions show that genomic selection is expected to yield a rapid reduction of mortality due to feather pecking, but a challenge will be to reduce mortality due to feather pecking in large groups.

INTRODUCTION

Mortality due to feather pecking (FP) is a worldwide problem, occurring in all kinds of commercial housing systems (Blokhuis and Arkes, 1984). Mortality due to FP has economic and welfare consequences for the commercial laying hen industry. FP is multifactorial and, among other factors, the occurrence of FP in

*esther.ellen@wur.nl

the laying period is influenced by rearing, light level in the barn, nutrition, group size and density, genotype and the effect of group members (Kjaer and Sorensen, 2002; Van Krimpen *et al.*, 2005; Ellen *et al.*, 2008). Furthermore, legislation has a large impact on the occurrence of FP. Due to the prohibition of the traditional battery cages in the European Union and the expected ban on beak trimming in many European countries in the near future, it is expected that mortality due to FP will increase. There is an urgent need to develop methods to reduce injurious FP in laying hens.

At first glance, selection against mortality due to FP should ideally be based on behavioural observations. Kjaer *et al.* (2001) used number of bouts of FP to select against FP behaviour. Unfortunately, collection of behavioural observations is time consuming, making breeding based on behavioural observations not feasible in practice. Moreover, behavioural observations often focus on the peckers only and ignore effects of the victim, and therefore yield a suboptimal response to selection (Ellen *et al.*, 2014a). Breeders need better solutions. A solution can come from quantitative genetic methods.

Mortality due to FP depends on social interactions between group members. With social interactions, the phenotype of an individual depends on its own genotype (direct genetic effect or victim effect) (DGE) and on the genotype of its group mates (indirect genetic effect or actor effect) (IGE). For survival time, we found that the victim effect contributes 13–64% of the total heritable variation, while the actor effect contributes 36–87% of the total heritable variation. Together, they explain 15–26% of total phenotypic variation in survival time (Ellen *et al.*, 2008; Peeters *et al.*, 2012). To select against mortality due to FP it is important to use a selection method that takes into account the effect of both the victim and the actor.

In animal breeding, genomic selection has become the method to genetically improve complex traits (Meuwissen *et al.*, 2001; Goddard and Hayes, 2009). Genomic selection is most useful for traits that are difficult to measure, cannot be measured on selection candidates (SC), cannot be measured on an individual before the breeding age, or have a low heritability (h^2) (Meuwissen *et al.*, 2001; Muir, 2007). Therefore, using genomic selection can be a promising tool to reduce mortality due to FP in laying hens.

The aim of this chapter is to present genetic solutions to reduce injurious FP in laying hens. It will present the results of a selection experiment using selection based on relatives, which takes into account the effect of the actor and victim (Ellen *et al.*, 2007). Furthermore, it will discuss the benefits of using genomic selection to reduce injurious FP in laying hens.

SELECTION METHOD

Muir (1996) showed that group selection can be used to select against mortality due to FP. Using group selection, mortality reduced from 68% to 8.8% in five generations (Muir, 1996). However, group selection is difficult to apply in the breeding of commercial laying hens, because SC should be housed in groups. When SC are housed in groups, it is difficult to record individual egg production;

therefore, in commercial breeding, a selection method is needed where SC are housed individually and selected based on the survival of relatives kept in family groups. Ellen *et al.* (2007) proposed the use of selection based on relatives, where SC are housed individually and selected based on the performance of siblings (sibs) or offspring with intact beaks kept in family groups.

Ellen *et al.* (2013, 2014a) performed a selection experiment against mortality due to FP using selection based on relatives. In total, six generations were selected. In each generation, individually housed SC were selected based on the average survival time of relatives kept in family groups. Relatives had intact beaks and were kept with four or five birds in traditional battery cages (Ellen *et al.*, 2014a). For generations 1, 5, and 6, SC were selected in two directions: high and low survival. Remaining SC were used to breed a control group. For generations 2, 3 and 4, SC were selected only to breed high survival and there was no control present (Ellen *et al.*, 2014a). Hens of the six generations were kept at different locations. Therefore, it was not possible to compare hens of the high survival line across generations. Figure 4.1 shows the survival percentage across generations.

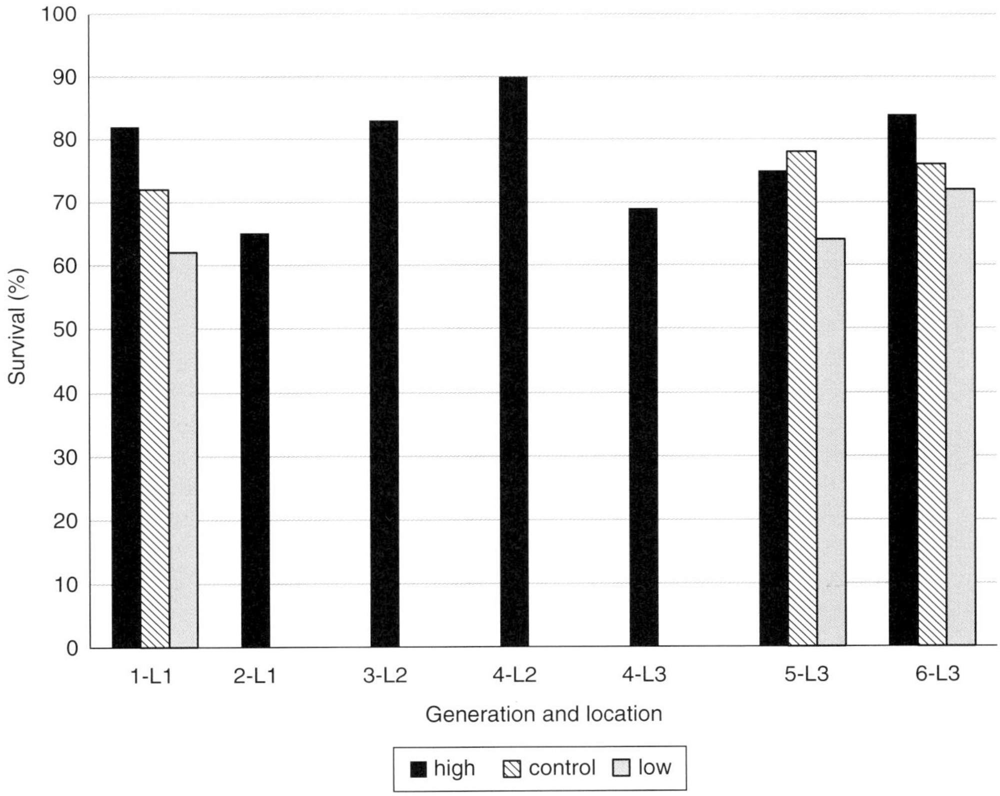

Fig. 4.1. Survival (%) for high survival, control and low survival groups in six generations at different locations (L1, L2, L3). In L1, hens of generations 1 and 2 were kept in a different barn at the same location.

Ellen *et al.* (2014a) showed the expected and realized responses for generations 1, 5 and 6. Expected responses were small, because selection intensity was small. This was due to the fact that SC were selected at 55 weeks of age, when there was limited variation in survival time. In generations 1, 5 and 6, the realized difference in survival days between high survival and low survival ranged from 26 to 29 days. Difference in survival days between high survival and control was 13 and 19 days in generations 1 and 6, respectively, whereas the difference was −12 days in generation 5. On average, these realized differences agreed with the theoretical expectation (Ellen *et al.*, 2014a). These results show that selection against mortality due to FP is feasible under ordinary commercial circumstances, but also that it is difficult to achieve high intensities of selection. Furthermore, Fig. 4.1 shows that survival is very sensitive to changes in the environment.

BREEDING PROGRAMMES

In commercial poultry breeding, SC are housed individually and selected based on own performance or on performance of sibs or offspring kept in family groups (also known as recurrent testing) (RT). Ellen *et al.* (2014a) showed that, using the RT design, it is possible to select against mortality due to FP. However, response to selection was small (Ellen *et al.*, 2014b). This is mainly because: (i) survival time is only known at the end of the laying period and censoring is high, i.e. many hens are still alive at the end of the laying period; and (ii) for SC, own performance records on survival time under field conditions (measured in multiple bird groups) are not available. Therefore information for sibs or offspring of the SC is used, which leads to limited accuracy of selection and long generation interval (when using offspring). To overcome this, genomic selection might offer solutions.

E.D. Ellen and P. Bijma (2017, unpublished results) compared a classical RT design, currently used to select against mortality due to FP, with two genomic selection designs: (i) only males are genotyped; and (ii) both males and females are genotyped. For the different breeding programmes, response to selection was compared. Prediction of response to selection was done using the SELACTION software (Rutten *et al.*, 2002). SELACTION accounts for the 'Bulmer effect', i.e. reduction in variance due to selection (Bulmer, 1971; Bijma, 2012). This is important for the classical RT design, because accuracies differ substantially between sexes (Dekkers, 1992; Bijma, 2012; Gorjanc *et al.*, 2015). Table 4.1 gives an overview of the parameters of the different breeding programmes, as implemented in SELACTION. A part of the parameters was taken from Alemu *et al.* (2016). More details about the different selection designs are given below.

Classical RT design

For the classical RT design, crossbred laying hens are kept in sire-family groups to test the sires. The sires are known, whereas the dams are unknown. Males are

Table 4.1. Input parameters[a] used in SELACTION to estimate response to selection for the different breeding programmes.

		Genomic selection	
	Classical RT	Males	Males and females
Selected proportion males	8%	2%	2%
Selected proportion females	8%	8%	8%
Generation interval males	99 weeks	33 weeks	33 weeks
Generation interval females	55 weeks	55 weeks	38 weeks
Information used for males	Progeny (80)	Own[b]	Own[b]
Information used for females	Sibs	Sibs	Own[b]
Number of sires (dams)	20 (400)	20 (400)	20 (400)

[a]Input parameters are based on Alemu *et al.* (2016). [b]Own means that SC are genotyped.

selected based on pedigree information and on the average phenotype of crossbred offspring (progeny testing), whereas females are selected based on pedigree information only (Alemu *et al.*, 2016). Female SC do not have own performance on survival in group housing, because SC are housed individually. Furthermore, information on survival of sibs is limited at time of selection, because there is limited variation in survival. Males are usually selected when they are almost 2 years of age, females are selected when they are approximately 1 year of age (Table 4.1) (Alemu *et al.*, 2016). In the RT design, groups consist of paternal sibs. Therefore, selection for ordinary estimated breeding values (EBV) captures the total breeding value (σ^2_{TBV}) for survival time, including both the DGE and IGE (Peeters, 2015).

Genomic selection designs

For the simulation of the genomic selection (GS) designs, the approach of Schrooten *et al.* (2005) and Dekkers (2007) was used. An additional correlated trait with full heritability was added, which represents the marker information. The genetic correlation (r_a) between the marker information and survival time can be determined based on the accuracy of the genomic estimated total breeding value (GETBV). The accuracy (ρ_{GS}) depends on the level of linkage disequilibrium (LD) between markers and the level of family relationships (Daetwyler *et al.*, 2008). Using the Daetwyler equation, the accuracy of GS (ρ_{GS}) was predicted to be 0.61 for survival time (E.D. Ellen and P. Bijma, 2017, unpublished results). The generation interval using genomic selection was 33 weeks for males and 38 weeks for females. The genotyped SC are selected based on the GETBV.

Response to selection

Table 4.2 shows the predicted accuracy and response to selection using the different breeding programmes. With the classical RT design, survival time can be

Table 4.2. Predicted accuracy and response to selection for the different breeding programmes selecting for survival time.

		Genomic selection	
	Classical RT	Males	Males and females
Accuracy males	0.85	0.54	0.49
Accuracy females	0.17	0.09	0.49
Response to selection (days/generation)	39.58	33.40	46.14
Response to selection (days/year)	26.73	39.48	67.59

Inputs for SELACTION are in Table 4.1; additional inputs: $\hat{\sigma}_p^2 = 13890$ days^2 and $T^2 = 0.17$ (E.D. Ellen and P. Bijma, 2017, unpublished results). For the genomic selection designs, the genetic correlation between survival time and marker information (r_a) is 0.61. Corresponding phenotypic correlation $r_p = hr_a = 0.25$. Heritability marker information = 100%, and phenotypic variance marker information ($r_a^2 h^2 \sigma_p^2$) = 879 days^2.

improved by 27 days per year. Including genotype information of the sire yielded a 48% increase in response to selection for survival time. This is mainly due to the decrease in generation interval. Using genomic selection for both males and females yielded a 153% increase in response to selection for survival time compared with classical RT.

The theoretical predictions shown in Table 4.2 indicate that mortality due to FP can be reduced rapidly when using genomic information for both male and female SC. However, there are still some challenges when selecting against mortality due to FP in practice. These challenges are discussed below.

CHALLENGES

Group size

There is a trend towards keeping commercial laying hens in larger groups. When animals are kept in large groups, it is difficult to identify social interactions between group members and to identify both victims and actors of FP. Current developments in sensor technologies, such as ultra-wideband (UWB) tracking, video tracking or radio-frequency identification (RFID), make it possible to identify and follow animals in small groups (e.g. Quwaider *et al.*, 2010; Banerjee *et al.*, 2014; Siegford *et al.*, 2016). For small groups the sensors can be used to identify social interactions between group members and to identify victims and actors (Rodenburg *et al.*, 2017). Studies in research facilities show that it is possible to detect the location of a bird with an 85% accuracy using UWB tracking (Rodenburg *et al.*, 2017). When the location of birds can be monitored, it is possible to identify the individuals that potentially interact with each other, so that a model to estimate direct and indirect breeding values can be set up (the key component is the incidence matrix Zs of the indirect effects). However, this approach has not been developed yet, and the resulting accuracy of estimated total breeding values is unknown. Moreover, further development of sensor technology is needed to facilitate application under commercial circumstances (i.e. large group sizes and harsh environments).

Level of mortality

Table 4.2 shows that response to selection for survival time is substantial, which may suggest that we are able to eliminate mortality due to FP in only a few generations. However, when mortality decreases, heritability and phenotypic variance of survival time become smaller, so that response to selection will become much smaller. This phenomenon is illustrated by the low heritability of survival time in lines with little mortality (e.g. the WF-line) (Ellen *et al.*, 2008) and is also seen when selecting on a threshold trait (Dempster and Lerner, 1950). Hence, results in Table 4.2 relate to the first generation of response to selection. So far, the effect of level of mortality on response to selection for survival time has not been investigated to our knowledge. Further research is needed to investigate this effect and how to deal with this in breeding programmes. One solution could be to keep the genomic reference population in a challenging environment, so that it shows greater mortality and thus higher accuracy of ETBV, but this raises questions in relation to animal welfare.

Commercial breeding

In commercial breeding, selection is based on an index of multiple traits. In this study, the focus was on single trait selection. Selecting for multiple traits will reduce response in a single trait. Nevertheless, even with multiple traits, genomic selection will outperform the traditional RT designs. Our results show that it is in principle feasible to reduce mortality due to FP by genetic selection. It is a matter of choice of breeding goal whether such a reduction will be realized in practice. In other words, it depends on the weight that breeding companies give to mortality due to FP, relative to other traits.

In commercial breeding, the end product is a crossbred animal. This means that purebred SC are ideally selected based on information of crossbred relatives, or a crossbred reference population. Mortality due to FP tends to be larger in crossbreds than in purebreds (Ellen *et al.*, 2008; Peeters *et al.*, 2012). Furthermore, there can be a large difference in the level of mortality due to FP in different crossbred populations. Brinker *et al.* (2017) showed that survival of hens originating from four different dam lines and the same sire line varied from 63% to 78%. In another study, Peeters *et al.* (2012) showed that reciprocal crosses differed substantially in the level of mortality. Furthermore, they showed that the genetic correlation between DGE of the two crosses was high, whereas the genetic correlation of IGE was only moderate. These results indicate that it matters which line provides the sire and which provides the dam (Peeters *et al.*, 2012). Therefore, to select against mortality due to FP in crossbred laying hens, it is important to take into account the parent-of-origin effect. Moreover, when the genetic correlation between different crosses is only moderate, this will limit response to selection when a single purebred line is used to produce multiple crosses. In this context, there is scope for research on the optimum design of genomic selection breeding programmes.

CONCLUSION

Mortality due to FP is an important economic and welfare trait in the commercial laying hen industry. Genetic solutions can be used to reduce mortality due to FP. IGE contribute substantially to the total heritable variation in survival time. Therefore, it is important to use a selection method that takes both the direct (victim effect) and indirect (actor effect) genetic effect into account. Model predictions show that genomic selection can yield a rapid reduction of mortality due to FP. A challenge will be to reduce mortality due to FP in large groups. But the combination of new sensor technologies and genomic information will be a powerful approach to reduce mortality due to FP in large groups.

ACKNOWLEDGEMENT

We would like to thank the employees of the laying houses for taking care of hens and data collection on survival. Data of this research was part of a joint project of Hendrix Genetics and Wageningen University and Research. The study was financially supported by the Dutch Technology Foundation STW and the Dutch science council (NWO).

REFERENCES

Alemu, S.W., Calus, M.P.L., Muir, W.M., Peeters, K., Vereijken, A. and Bijma, P. (2016) Genomic prediction of survival time in a population of brown laying hens showing cannibalistic behavior. *Genetics Selection Evolution* 48, 68.

Banerjee, D., Daigle, C.L., Dong, B., Wurtz, K., Newberry, R.C., Siegford, J.M. and Biswas, S. (2014) Detection of jumping and landing force in laying hens using wireless wearable sensors. *Poultry Science* 93, 2724–2733.

Bijma, P. (2012) Accuracies of estimated breeding values from ordinary genetic evaluations do not reflect the correlation between true and estimated breeding values in selected populations. *Journal of Animal Breeding and Genetics* 129(5), 345–358.

Blokhuis, H.J. and Arkes, J.G. (1984) Some observations on the development of feather pecking in poultry. *Applied Animal Behaviour Science* 12, 145–157.

Brinker, T., Raymond, B., Bijma, P., Vereijken, A. and Ellen, E. (2017) Estimation of total genetic effects for survival time in crossbred laying hens showing cannibalism, using pedigree or genomic information. *Journal of Animal Breeding and Genetics* 134, 60–68.

Bulmer, M.G. (1971) Effect of selection on genetic variability. *The American Naturalist* 105(943), 201–211.

Daetwyler, H.D., Villanueva, B. and Woolliams, J.A. (2008) Accuracy of predicting the genetic risk of disease using a genome-wide approach. *PLOS ONE* 3(10), e3395.

Dekkers, J.C.M. (1992) Asymptotic response to selection on best linear unbiased predictors of breeding values. *Animal Production* 54(03), 351–360.

Dekkers, J.C.M. (2007) Prediction of response to marker-assisted and genomic selection using selection index theory. *Journal of Animal Breeding and Genetics* 124(6), 331–341.

Dempster, E.R. and Lerner, I.M. (1950) Heritability of threshold characters. *Genetics* 35, 212–236.

Ellen, E.D., Muir, W.M., Teuscher, F. and Bijma, P. (2007) Genetic improvement of traits affected by interactions among individuals: Sib selection schemes. *Genetics* 176, 489–499.

Ellen, E.D., Visscher, J., van Arendonk, J.A.M. and Bijma, P. (2008) Survival of laying hens: genetic parameters for direct and associative effects in three purebred layer lines. *Poultry Science* 87, 233–239.

Ellen, E.D., Rodenburg, T.B., Visscher, J. and Bijma, P. (2013) The consequence of selection on social genetic effects for survival in laying hens. *8th European Symposium on Poultry Genetics*, Venice, Italy. pp. 35–38.

Ellen, E.D., Rodenburg, T.B., Albers, G.A.A., Bolhuis, J.E., Camerlink, I. *et al.* , (2014a) The prospects of selection for social genetic effects to improve welfare and productivity in livestock. *Frontiers in Genetics* 5, 377.

Ellen, E.D., Visscher, J. and Bijma, P. (2014b) Comparison of empirical and theoretical responses to selection against mortality due to cannibalism in layers. *Proceedings of the10th World Conference on Genetics Applied to Livestock Production*, Vancouver, Abstract 317.

Goddard, M.E. and Hayes, B.J. (2009) Mapping genes for complex traits in domestic animals and their use in breeding programmes. *Nature Reviews Genetics* 10(6), 381–391.

Gorjanc, G., Bijma, P. and Hickey, J.M. (2015) Reliability of pedigree based and genomic evaluations in selected populations. *Genetics Selection Evolution* 47(1), 65.

Kjaer, J.B. and Sorensen, P. (2002) Feather pecking and cannibalism in free-range laying hens as affected by genotype, dietary level of methionine + cystine, light intensity during rearing and age at first access to the range area. *Applied Animal Behaviour Science* 76, 21–39.

Kjaer, J.B., Sorensen, P. and Su, G. (2001) Divergent selection on feather pecking behaviour in laying hens (*Gallus gallus domesticus*). *Applied Animal Behaviour Science* 71, 229–239.

Meuwissen, T.H.E., Hayes, B.J. and Goddard, M.E. (2001) Prediction of total genetic value using genome-wide dense marker maps. *Genetics* 157, 1819–1829.

Muir, W.M. (1996) Group selection for adaptation to multiple-hen cages: selection program and direct responses. *Poultry Science* 75, 447–458.

Muir, W.M. (2007) Comparison of genomic and traditional BLUP-estimated breeding value accuracy and selection response under alternative trait and genomic parameters. *Journal of Animal Breeding and Genetics* 124, 342–355.

Peeters, K., Eppink, T.T., Ellen, E.D., Visscher, J. and Bijma, P. (2012) Indirect genetic effects for survival in domestic chicken (*Gallus gallus*) are magnified in crossbred genotypes and show a parent-of-origin effect. *Genetics* 192, 705–713.

Peeters, K. (2015) Genetics of social interactions in laying hens: improving survival and productivity. PhD thesis, Wageningen University.

Quwaider, M., Daigle, C., Biswas, S., Siegford, J. and Swanson, J. (2010) Development of a wireless body-mounted sensor to monitor location and activity of laying hens in a non-cage housing system. *Transactions of the ASABE* 53, 1705–1713.

Rodenburg, T.B., Bennewitz, J., de Haas, E.N., Košťál, L., Pichová, K. *et al.* (2017) The Use of Sensor Technology and Genomics to Breed for Laying Hens That Show Less Damaging Behaviour. In: Berckmans, D. and Keita, A. (eds) *Precision Livestock Farming '17*. Papers presented at the 8th European Conference on Precision Livestock Farming, Nantes, France, 12–14 September 2017, pp. 532–541.

Rutten, M.J.M., Bijma, P., Woolliams, J.A. and Arendonk, J.A.M. (2002) SelAction: software to predict selection response and rate of inbreeding in livestock breeding programs. *Journal of Heredity* 93(6), 456–458.

Schrooten, C., Bovenhuis, H., Arendonk, J.A.M. and Bijma, P. (2005) Genetic progress in multistage dairy cattle breeding schemes using genetic markers. *Journal of Dairy Science* 88(4), 1569–1581.

Siegford, J.M., Berezowski, J., Biswas, S.K., Daigle, C. L., Gebhardt-Henrich, S.G., Hernandez, C.E., Thurner, S. and Toscano, M.J. (2016) Assessing activity and location of individual laying hens in large groups using modern technology. *Animals* 6(2), 10.

Van Krimpen, M.M., Kwakkel, R.P., Reuvekamp, B.F.J., Van Der Peet-Schwering, C.M.C., Den Hartog, L.A. and Verstegen, M.W.A. (2005) Impact of feeding management on feather pecking in laying hens. *World's Poultry Science Journal* 61(04), 663–686.

CHAPTER 5
Evidence-based Management of Injurious Pecking

Thea van Niekerk*

Wageningen Livestock Research, Wageningen, The Netherlands

ABSTRACT

Injurious pecking in laying hen flocks comprises feather pecking and tissue pecking, the latter often referred to as cannibalism. Although some gentle feather pecking belongs to the natural repertoire of laying hens, the more vigorous form, severe feather pecking, is considered an abnormal behaviour. Various theories have been developed to explain the onset of injurious pecking. All point to suboptimal circumstances leading to abnormal or redirected behaviour. A wide range of husbandry and management factors have been identified. They affect either the onset of injurious pecking (prevention) or its reduction. Prevention is most important, because once started the behaviour is very hard to stop. Therefore the first focus should be on optimizing rearing conditions to prevent injurious pecking. The most important management strategy in rear is a continuous presence of high-quality substrate to stimulate foraging behaviour and to allow the pullets to develop a habit of directing their pecking towards the litter. Any stressor can be a trigger for injurious pecking. This means management should also focus on the prevention of stressful events. Such stressful events may be changes in housing conditions (e.g. transition from rear to lay, climate) and management (e.g. light, feed, access to range), but also suboptimal health, especially parasites and compromised intestinal health. Finally some husbandry conditions seem to increase the propensity to develop injurious pecking, such as large flock sizes and a higher bird density. Management to prevent injurious pecking can only be successful if it aims at optimizing all factors involved.

*thea.vanniekerk@wur.nl

INTRODUCTION

Feather pecking (FP) and other forms of injurious pecking are behaviours with a complex background. Although there are some theories about the causation of FP behaviour, many of the underlying causes are still unknown, but there are various management strategies that appear successful in reducing the risk of FP.

Feather pecking is a serious problem. A survey among Swiss farmers indicated that one-third of farmers took action against FP (Huber-Eicher and Audige, 1999). In the UK 47% of the farmers considered FP a normal occurrence (Green *et al.*, 2000) and indicated that 65% of their flocks showed FP at some point (Nicol *et al.*, 2013). However, researchers found that FP in commercial flocks was occurring at a higher frequency than farmers themselves reported. They found signs of gentle FP in 89% of the observed flocks at the age of 25 weeks. At that age, in 69% of the flocks signs of severe FP were also found. At 40 weeks gentle FP dropped to 73%, but severe FP increased and occurred in 86% of the flocks (Lambton *et al.*, 2010). In another UK study, Gilani *et al.* (2013) found gentle FP in 94% of the flocks in both rear and lay; severe FP was observed in 27% of the rearing flocks and 65% of the layer flocks. In Sweden 62% of flocks were affected by FP (Gunnarsson *et al.*, 1999). This indicates that the problem is very widespread.

Feather pecking does not always cause feather damage. Gentle feather pecking (GFP) comprises repeated gentle pecking or licking at the tips and edges of feathers. It is usually ignored by the recipient (Savory, 1995). GFP is commonly regarded as not harmful to the feathers. However, if the pecking starts to become more severe it may harm the feathers or cause feathers to be pulled out. This is commonly referred to as severe feather pecking (SFP). Rodenburg *et al.* (2013) used the following definition for severe feather pecking: 'It consists of forceful pecks and pulls of feathers that are frequently eaten and results in feather loss on the back, vent and tail area. Victims of SFP often initially show a behavioural response to receiving SFP, either by moving away or by confronting the pecker. If SFP continues, however, victims have also been observed to surrender to being pecked and remain still.' Although scientists continue to debate whether there is a relationship between GFP and SFP (Rodenburg *et al.*, 2004b; Lambton *et al.*, 2010), in practice GFP in the laying period is usually regarded as a first warning signal for the start of SFP.

In this chapter an overview is given of possible management strategies that may prevent the start of FP or could help to control or reduce this behaviour.

FEATHER DAMAGE

Feather damage is not always due to pecking. Feathers from the breast and front of the neck can deteriorate due to frequent contact with the feeder. The back of the neck can have rough feather cover due to moulting. Wing feathers can be damaged by the housing system, especially wire side partitions. Bellies of high-producing hens are often bald due to sitting and rubbing on the artificial mat in the nest boxes. Also tail feathers can be damaged by the system. Feather damage on these body parts due to FP cannot be excluded, but one should be aware that feather wear may have other causes than FP.

Monitoring the occurrence of FP is mostly done by monitoring feather damage. For this, often only those body parts where feather damage is most clearly related to feather pecking are scored. Therefore in pullets only the neck, back, tail base, tail, cloaca region and wing feathers are scored. In laying hens the neck, back, tail base and cloaca region are scored. The front of the neck, wings and belly mostly are not scored as feather damage in those regions may have other causes than FP. For both pullets and laying hens the back of the head is only scored in relation to aggression, not in relation to feather pecking.

CONSEQUENCES OF FEATHER PECKING

Feather pecking with feather damage as a result has some more adverse effects. Due to feather loss the insulation of the feather cover reduces, causing heat loss. This leads to an increase in feed consumption, which may be as high as 40% (Blokhuis *et al.*, 2007). Feather pecking may also escalate into cannibalism and consequently into increased mortality. In furnished cages mortality is usually low, but it may increase up to 65% due to injurious pecking (Weitzenburger *et al.*, 2005). In non-cage systems mortality levels are very variable and can run up to 20–30%, of which 6–26% is due to cannibalism (Rodenburg *et al.*, 2012; Nicol *et al.*, 2013). Apart from the direct effects of injurious pecking, there is also an indirect effect. Birds that are pecked at will experience stress, which increases the risk for various diseases (Nicol *et al.*, 2013).

BEAK TRIMMING VERSUS NOT TRIMMING

The most applied preventive measure against injurious feather pecking is beak trimming. However, as this procedure is painful, even if it is done with infrared, and negatively affects the tactile senses of the beak permanently, it is seen as an unwanted procedure in terms of animal welfare and the intrinsic value of the animal (Glatz, 2005; Kuenzel, 2007; Jongman *et al.*, 2008; Marchant-Forde *et al.*, 2008). Beak trimming does reduce the effect of injurious pecking, but it does not prevent or reduce the behaviour itself (Glatz, 2005; Lambton *et al.*, 2013). Recently more and more countries have been banning the practice of routine beak trimming. Also the demand for eggs from intact flocks is increasing, resulting in more farmers keeping intact flocks. We recently made an inventory among four Dutch hatching/rearing companies to compare mortality levels between layer flocks that had been beak trimmed and those that were not. In total the inventory comprised 259 trimmed flocks and 81 untrimmed flocks in the period 2013–2016. The average mortality of the untrimmed flocks was higher at all ages compared to the mortality of the trimmed flocks (personal data, not published). With ageing of the flocks the difference in mortality gradually increased until the average cumulative mortality of the untrimmed flocks was 1.8% higher than in the trimmed flocks at 80 weeks of age. The overall mortality of the untrimmed and trimmed flocks at 85 weeks of age, averaged over all systems and genotypes, was 8% and 6%, respectively.

DOES MANAGEMENT HELP?

Management is important to both prevent and treat or reduce injurious pecking behaviour. This was confirmed in a trial on commercial farms conducted by Lambton *et al.* (2013). The authors carried out a systematic review of scientific literature and generated 46 potentially protective management strategies. They designed management packages for 53 treatment flocks (TF) on 47 farms. On average the farmers applied 21 management strategies. For 47 control flocks (on 44 farms) no management advice was given. On average the farmers with control flocks applied 17 management strategies. All flocks were scored on feather cover and feather pecking behaviour at 20, 30 and 40 weeks of age. The results indicated that if more management strategies were applied, there was less FP, a better feather cover and a lower mortality at 40 weeks of age. Thus, good management can indeed lower the risk of FP.

FACTORS AFFECTING THE ONSET OF FEATHER PECKING

Feather pecking is thought to result from the inability to perform normal foraging behaviour (Blokhuis, 1986). In the absence of adequate foraging material the birds seek another substrate, which often includes the feathers of conspecifics. Also the inability to perform normal dust-bathing behaviour has been mentioned as a cause for injurious pecking behaviour (Vestergaard *et al.*, 1997). Besides these basic causes of feather pecking related to litter quality (for foraging and/or for dust bathing), there are many more factors known to influence the start, development and extent of injurious pecking. Figure 5.1 shows the factors grouped in a schedule. Various elements in the environment of the bird influence the possible onset of FP. These factors are related to management, housing, feeding, etc. Also, properties of the animal itself contribute to the risk for FP. These animal-based properties concern fairly fixed factors like genetics and parental influences, but also some more variable factors like hormonal status and health status. Figure 5.1 includes only those factors confirmed in research, but not all factors are equally well investigated and also little is known about the interactions between factors. Figure 5.1 is not intended to give a precise model for the onset of FP; it merely serves to illustrate the complexity of the problem. Also it emphasizes that FP cannot be solved by focusing on one factor; it should focus on acquiring a balance in all influencing factors. When, for some reason, the balance is disturbed, normal behaviour will evolve into problem behaviour.

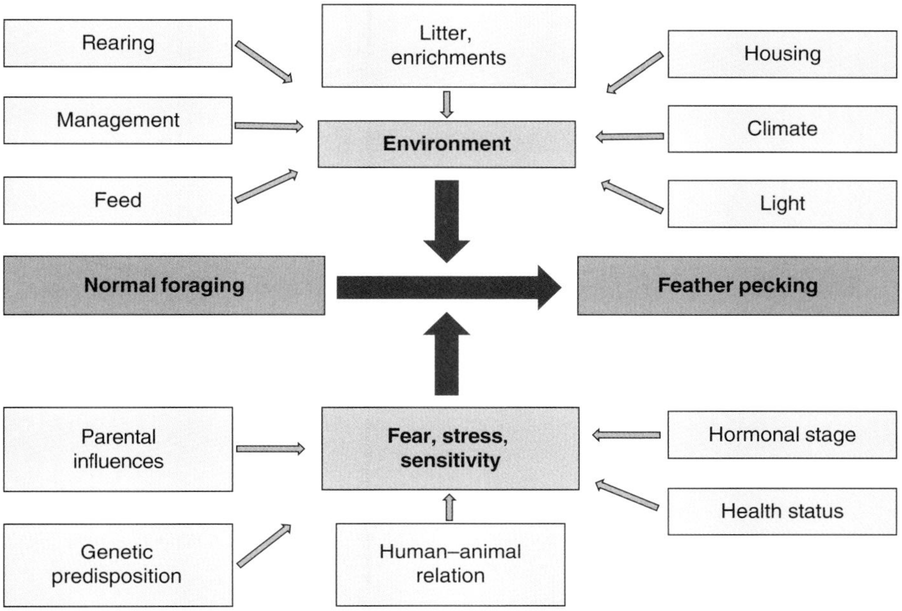

Fig. 5.1. Influences on the onset of feather pecking.

Genetic background of feather pecking

Genotypes differ in their predisposition to start FP. Divergent selection for high and low FP resulted in significant differences in FP behaviour and plumage condition (Kjaer and Hocking, 2004). Various studies have indicated a relationship between fearfulness and FP, where more fearful lines tend to perform more FP (Rodenburg *et al.*, 2010).

De Haas *et al.* (2014) found a relationship between the level of anxiety of the parent stock and SFP in the offspring. In white genotypes, but not in brown, more stressed parent stock produced offspring that were more prone to perform SFP. In brown genotypes the environmental factors were more important. The authors also found a relationship between disruption and limitation of litter supply at an early age and SFP, feather damage and fearfulness in the laying period for brown genotypes, but not for white genotypes. This indicates that genetic factors may affect a bird's sensitivity to certain risk factors for FP.

Rearing conditions

Many researchers found that rearing in a proper way is one of the most important measures to prevent FP. Bestman *et al.* (2009a) monitored FP in 28 rearing flocks that later were split up over 51 layer houses. They recorded FP both in rear and in lay and found high correlations between the incidence of FP in rear and in lay. Where there was no FP in rear, there was a 71% chance that the layer flock would not perform FP. Where there was FP in rear already, there was a 90% chance that the hens would continue this behaviour in the laying period.

De Haas and Rodenburg (2014) found high levels of FP in the rearing period at around 5 weeks of age. At this age the birds often experience a disruption of litter, which coincides with one of the moulting stages. The authors found a strong correlation between FP at 5 weeks of age and high levels of feather damage at 40 weeks of age. Flocks in which specific management to prevent FP and fearfulness was applied (radio, pecking blocks) had less feather damage at 40 weeks of age compared with flocks with standard management. These findings strongly suggest that management aimed at reducing FP should start early in the rearing period.

At the end of the rearing period the pullets are transported to the layer units. To make this transition as smooth as possible farmers should put effort into reducing stress and have as much as possible the same housing and management in the layer unit as in rear (temperature, light, feed) (Van de Weerd and Elson, 2006; De Jong *et al.*, 2013.

Fearfulness

Many studies found a relationship between fearfulness and feather pecking (Rodenburg *et al.*, 2013). Rodenburg *et al.* (2004a) found that if birds were fearful as chicks they were more likely to develop feather pecking as adults.

A low FP line responded less fearfully in an open field than a high FP line (Jones *et al.*, 1995). Although Rodenburg *et al.* (2010) could not find differences in fearfulness between lines divergently selected for FP, they did emphasize the relationship between FP and fear: 'While fear can be increased due to FP, increased fearfulness can also be a predictor for the development of FP.' Fearful birds may be more sensitive to on-farm stressors like management procedures, feed changes and unexpected events. Therefore management to reduce fearfulness may reduce the risk for FP.

One way to reduce fearfulness is to reduce the birds' fear of humans. If birds are less fearful of humans they will be less flighty, which will also lead to fewer casualties and possibly to better production (Hemsworth, 2004). Palczynski *et al.* (2016) and Hemsworth (2009) emphasized the importance of stockperson education, not only regarding their knowledge of keeping hens, but also regarding their attitude and behaviour towards animals. Habituation of birds to humans can be achieved by having various people taking care of the birds, wearing different clothing, variation in daily routines, playing a radio and talking to the birds. Other ways to calm the birds are habits like walking calmly, giving birds time to move away and knocking on the door before entering the house.

Hormonal status

FP in the production period starts to show around 40–50 weeks of age. Upon closer inspection, it seems that often FP has already commenced at the start of lay or even earlier (Lambton *et al.*, 2010; De Haas and Rodenburg, 2014). As FP is often related to stress, the change from the rearing house to the layer unit and the physiological stress of the changing hormonal state due to the start of egg laying could be triggers for hens to start feather pecking.

Health

Health problems cause stress, which may be a trigger for hens to start FP. Health problems can have various causes, such as parasites and bacterial infections. Examples of parasites are red mites and worms. Red mites are prevalent in hen houses and can cause substantial irritation, leading to FP, and a strong infestation can cause anaemia, leading to reduced health and even mortality. The mites can also be a vector for viruses and bacteria (Valiente Moro *et al.*, 2009).

Worms can lead to reduced health due to reduced feed utilization, possibly leading to deficiencies. Worms can also influence the behaviour of hens negatively, leading to more agonistic behaviour and thus possibly also to more injurious pecking (Gauly *et al.*, 2007). Another health problem is *Escherichia coli*, which can cause substantial mortality (Selvam *et al.*, 2004). It is actually a so-called secondary infection, meaning that there is an underlying cause that weakened the birds and made them susceptible for *E. coli*. This may be another infection, such as infectious bronchitis (IB), but it can also be a stressor such as excessive FP. *E. coli* itself can also be the stressor that causes FP. Intestinal problems like *E. coli* can cause reduced feed utilization, leading to deficiencies and consequently a higher risk for FP (Van Krimpen *et al.*, 2005).

Nutrition

Nutrition plays a very important role in relation to FP (Van Krimpen *et al.*, 2005). This chapter will not go into details of the nutritional factors but a few general comments are presented. In general, feeding mash will reduce the risk for FP compared with feeding pellets (Aerni *et al.*, 2000; Lambton *et al.*, 2015). However, pelleted feed does not have the issue of segregation of ingredients, which also is very important, as nutritional imbalances may lead to FP. A lot is known about deficiencies causing FP, but much less is known about the correct feed composition to prevent FP. Van Krimpen *et al.* (2009) looked at the rearing and laying phase and concluded that (lower) energy concentration, (higher) non-starch polysaccharide (NSP) concentration and (larger) particle sizes of NSPs are favourable in preventing or postponing FP. Insoluble dietary fibre decreases the passage rate through the gut and therefore increase satiety.

Other important nutritional components are proteins. SFP increased when levels of crude protein were lower than 125 g/kg, lysine was lower than 8.2 g/kg or methionine and cysteine together were lower than 5.1 g/kg (Lambton *et al.*, 2015). In a large survey Green *et al.* (2000) found that more than three diet changes increased the risk of FP. Gilani *et al.* (2013) indicated that each diet change during rear resulted in a high risk of FP later in life. Diet changes as are done in phase feeding are necessary to adapt the feed to the needs of the birds. Also diet changes may result from providing a new batch of feed. As long as these diet changes take place gradually, probably no harmful effects will be caused. Nutritionists will have to find ways to make necessary diet changes as subtle as possible.

Since FP is probably (a form of) redirected ground pecking, directing the behaviour to the ground should reduce the risk for FP. In addition to keeping the litter dry and friable, providing roughage is a good way to stimulate foraging behaviour. Roughage should already be given in the rearing period. It is most effective if it contains edible particles (Van Krimpen *et al.*, 2005). Other objects that can direct pecking to the floor include pecking blocks, which also help to blunt the beaks and to keep the hens occupied.

Housing system

An accessible system, where birds can move around easily without the need to make large or steep jumps, facilitates the birds in moving around, finding food, water and nest boxes, and escaping from other birds in case of conflicts. Nest boxes are frequently equipped with dim lights to attract birds. Especially with hens laying eggs before the lights switch on in the henhouse, this can be a good management procedure to attract these hens to the nest box and thus prevent floor eggs and reduce the risk of vent pecking. However, the nest lights may also pose a risk for vent pecking (Potzsch *et al.*, 2001); therefore the lights should be switched off as much as possible. A good positioning of lights on the ceiling, so that some light enters the nest box, can make nest-box lights unnecessary.

Functional zones can be a good way to create resting areas where needed and activity where it should be. Experiences on commercial farms are positive and indicate a reduction in stress and aggression, possibly resulting in less FP (Donaldson and O'Connell, 2012). Functional zones can be foraging areas, where there is litter, food, roughage and a little more light to stimulate foraging behaviour. Resting zones comprise perches, preferably on an elevated place (top level of the aviary or on an A-frame). Nesting zones and resting zones should be a little dimmer to create a quiet place, but not too dim, as this could make it more difficult for hens to jump on to the perches (Moinard *et al.*, 2004). Positioning of perches properly should prevent vent pecking (Lambton *et al.*, 2015). This means that they should be placed either very low or high enough to prevent vent pecking (i.e. out of reach of conspecifics).

Gunnarsson *et al.* (1999) found that introduction of perches at 4 weeks of age reduced the risk of FP. Lambton *et al.* (2010) found less FP when perches were present in the laying period. In addition to the indoor area of the housing system, access to an outdoor range can reduce the risk for FP (Bestman and Wagenaar, 2003; Lambton *et al.*, 2010). This will specifically be the case if the range is used well. Main factors contributing to optimum use of the range are cover on the range (either artificial or bushes and trees), foraging possibilities (vegetation) and smaller flock sizes (Nagle and Glatz, 2012; Gebhardt-Henrich *et al.*, 2014). The presence of other animals (e.g. sheep, cows) may stimulate hens to join them in the outdoor use (Bestman *et al.*, 2009b). The presence of other animals also forms a protection from predators.

Stocking density and group size

Various studies have focused on stocking density and group size, but these factors are often confounded and also influenced by the type of housing. As a consequence, these factors are still poorly understood (Widowski *et al.*, 2016; Keeling *et al.*, 2017). Practical experience indicates that a lower density will often decrease FP. Free-range access offers extra space, which effectively reduces indoor stocking density. It also provides additional foraging possibilities, which may be the reason why increased free-range use is associated with reduced FP damage (Lambton *et al.*, 2010; Nicol *et al.*, 2013). In general smaller group sizes are favourable in preventing FP, as is the case in furnished cages, where feather damage due to FP usually is lower compared with non-cage systems (Nicol *et al.*, 2013).

Air quality

Air quality and temperature can have an influence on the onset of FP. Suboptimal environmental temperatures (either high or low) and high ammonia (NH_3) levels are a risk for FP (Lambton *et al.*, 2010; Nicol *et al.*, 2013). The air in poultry houses usually contains high dust levels, which may affect health of the birds (Matkovic *et al.*, 2009). Pop-holes may cause draughts and this may challenge the health of the birds. Each health challenge puts stress on the birds and therefore implies a risk for the onset of FP. Not much is known about the effects of noise on stress and welfare of hens. High noise levels could cause more stress.

Light may affect stress levels of laying hens. There are many aspects of light that can influence the birds, like length of the light period, light intensity, light distribution, spectrum of the light and light source (Lewis and Morris, 2006).

Fluorescent light (FL) sources produce a flickering light. The flickering of low-frequency FL can be detected by the birds and cause stress and thus is a risk for FP (Prescott *et al.*, 2004). Recently light sources in many hen houses have been replaced by light-emitting diode (LED) lights. Although these are known to have a flat current, there may be flickering that can be seen by hens, caused by the software in the dimming equipment (Lisney *et al.*, 2011). It is often suggested that light intensity should be low to prevent FP (Mohammed *et al.*, 2010). At low light intensities birds cannot see wounds and thus do not peck at them. However, low light intensities also make the hens more fearful, possibly causing more FP. A lot is still unknown about light preferences and effects of lights (Prescott *et al.*, 2004). Some results are contradictory. For instance, some studies indicate adverse effects of daylight on FP, while other studies suggest the opposite. We found less FP when more unfiltered daylight was present, and more FP when (more) filtered daylight was present (T. van Niekerk, unpublished data). Windows act as a filter. As a result the light no longer contains ultraviolet (UV) wavelengths.

As birds can see UV (Lewis and Gous, 2009), these two types of daylight are perceived differently, possibly explaining the effects on FP.

Management

As discussed earlier, applying measures to prevent and reduce FP does have effects (Lambton *et al.*, 2013). Management to prevent FP should aim at reducing risk factors in feeding, housing, control and treatment of the flock (Van de Weerd and Elson, 2006; Thiele and Pottguter, 2008; Lambton *et al.*, 2010; Nicol *et al.*, 2013; Heerkens *et al.*, 2015; Janczak and Riber, 2015). Frequent flock walks are not only recommended for early detection of FP problems, but may also result in less fear of humans. Regarding management, farmers should pay extra attention to climate, climate changes, disease problems (intestinal problems, infections, parasites), frequent removal of eggs laid on floor, dead and wounded birds (cannibalism). Also unexpected events should be prevented as much as possible, as they may pose a considerable stress on the birds.

Finally, economics plays an important role in making management decisions. Farmers tend to make decisions on saving cost. However, within reasonable limits spending extra money can result in better zootechnical results, less FP and thus a higher income. Experiences of farmers with flocks with intact beaks indicate that good-quality feed may be more expensive, but reduces the risk and extent of FP and thus may in the end give a higher yield. The same effect can be expected of a good rearing environment. Both in rear and in lay, use of roughages or pecking blocks may result in better feather cover, and thus lower feed costs.

CONCLUSIONS

This chapter has presented a wide range of factors influencing the onset of FP. Each of these factors may contribute to the overall risk for FP. Not much is known about their interaction, but it is known that none of these factors in itself is sufficient to control FP. Reducing the overall risk for FP means minimizing at least a number of possible causes, if not all of them.

REFERENCES

Aerni, V., El-Lethey, H. and Wechsler, B. (2000) Effect of foraging material and food form on feather pecking in laying hens. *British Poultry Science* 41, 16–21.

Bestman, M.W.P. and Wagenaar, J.P. (2003) Farm level factors associated with feather pecking in organic laying hens. *Livestock Production Science* 80, 133–140.

Bestman, M., Koene, P. and Wagenaar, J.P. (2009a) Influence of farm factors on the occurrence of feather pecking in organic reared hens and their predictability for feather pecking in the laying period. *Applied Animal Behaviour Science* 121, 120–125.

Bestman, M., Loefs, R., Vries, H.D. and Van De Burgt, G.-J. (2009b) *Kippenuitloop Gezond en Groen; Inspiratie en ideeën voor ontwerp en uitvoering*. LBI publication LV74. Louis Bolk Institute , Driebergen, The Netherlands.

Blokhuis, H.J. (1986) Feather-pecking in poultry: its relation with ground-pecking. *Applied Animal Behaviour Science* 16, 63–67.

Blokhuis, H.J., Fiks van Niekerk, T.G.C.M., Bessei, W., Elson, H.A., Guémené, D. *et al.* (2007) The LayWel project: welfare implications of changes in production systems for laying hens. *World's Poultry Science Journal* 63, 101–114.

De Haas, E.N. and Rodenburg, T.B. (2014) Feather pecking in laying hens during rearing and laying in non-cage systems, management practices and farmers opinions. In: *Proceedings of the 48th Congress of the International Society for Applied Ethology (ISAE)*. Wageningen Academic Publishers, Wageningen, The Netherlands, p. 159.

De Haas, E.N., Bolhuis, J.E., Kemp, B., Groothuis, T.G.G. and Rodenburg, T.B. (2014) Parents and early life environment affect behavioral development of laying hen chickens. *PLOS ONE* 9, e90577.

De Jong, I.C., Rodenburg, T.B. and van Niekerk, T.G.C.M. (2013) Management approaches to reduce feather pecking in laying hens. *CAB Reviews: Perspectives in Agriculture, Veterinary Science, Nutrition and Natural Resources* 8, 1–8.

Donaldson, C.J. and O'Connell, N.E. (2012) The influence of access to aerial perches on fearfulness, social behaviour and production parameters in free-range laying hens. *Applied Animal Behaviour Science* 142, 51–60.

Gauly, M., Duss, C. and Erhardt, G. (2007) Influence of *Ascaridia galli* infections and anthelmintic treatments on the behaviour and social ranks of laying hens (*Gallus gallus domesticus*). *Veterinary Parasitology* 146, 271–280.

Gebhardt-Henrich, S.G., Toscano, M.J. and Fröhlich, E.K.F. (2014) Use of outdoor ranges by laying hens in different sized flocks. *Applied Animal Behaviour Science* 155, 74–81.

Gilani, A.-M., Knowles, T.G. and Nicol, C.J. (2013) The effect of rearing environment on feather pecking in young and adult laying hens. *Applied Animal Behaviour Science* 148, 54–63.

Glatz, P.C. (2005) *Poultry Welfare Issues – Beak Trimming.* Nottingham University Press, Nottingham, UK.

Green, L.E., Lewis, K., Kimpton, A. and Nicol, C.J. (2000) Cross-sectional study of the prevalence of feather pecking in laying hens in alternative systems and its associations with management and disease. *Veterinary Record* 147, 233–238.

Gunnarsson, S., Keeling, L.J. and Svedberg, J. (1999) Effect of rearing factors on the prevalence of floor eggs, cloacal cannibalism and feather pecking in commercial flocks of loose housed laying hens. *British Poultry Science* 40, 12–18.

Heerkens, J.L.T., Delezie, E., Kempen, I., Zoons, J., Ampe, B., Rodenburg, T.B. and Tuyttens, F.A.M. (2015) Specific characteristics of the aviary housing system affect plumage condition, mortality and production in laying hens. *Poultry Science* 94, 2008–2017.

Hemsworth, P.H. (2004) Human–animal interactions. In: Perry, G.C. (ed.) *Welfare of the Laying Hen*. CAB International, Wallingford, UK, pp. 329–343.

Hemsworth, P.H. (2009) Impact of human–animal interactions on the health, productivity and welfare of farm animals. In: Aland, A. and Madec, F. (eds) *Sustainable Animal Production*. Wageningen Academic Publishers, Wageningen, pp. 57–68.

Huber-Eicher, B. and Audige, L. (1999) Analysis of risk factors for the occurrence of feather pecking in laying hen growers. *British Poultry Science* 40, 599–604.

Janczak, A.M. and Riber, A.B. (2015) Review of rearing-related factors affecting the welfare of laying hens. *Poultry Science* 94, 1454–1469.

Jones, R.B., Blokhuis, H.J. and Beuving, G. (1995) Open-field and tonic immobility responses in domestic chicks of two genetic lines differing in their propensity to feather peck. *British Poultry Science* 36, 525–530.

Jongman, E.C., Glatz, P.C. and Barnett, J L. (2008) Changes in behaviour of laying hens following beak trimming at hatch and re-trimming at 14 weeks. *Asian-Australasian Journal of Animal Sciences* 21, 291–298.

Keeling, L.J., Newberry, R.C. and Estevez, I. (2017) Flock size during rearing affects pullet behavioural synchrony and spatial clustering. *Applied Animal Behaviour Science* 194, 36–41.

Kjaer, J.B. and Hocking, P.M. (2004) The genetics of feather pecking and cannibalism. In: Perry, G.C. (ed.) *Welfare of the Laying Hen.* CAB International, Wallingford, UK, pp. 109–121.

Kuenzel, W.J. (2007) Neurobiological basis of sensory perception: welfare implications of beak trimming. *Poultry Science* 86, 1273–1282.

Lambton, S.L., Knowles, T.G., Yorke, C. and Nicol, C.J. (2010) The risk factors affecting the development of gentle and severe feather pecking in loose housed laying hens. *Applied Animal Behaviour Science* 123, 32–42.

Lambton, S.L., Nicol, C.J., Friel, M., Main, D.C.J., McKinstry, J.L. *et al.* (2013) A bespoke management package can reduce levels of injurious pecking in loose-housed laying hen flocks. *Veterinary Record* 172, 423.

Lambton, S.L., Knowles, T.G., Yorke, C. and Nicol, C.J. (2015) The risk factors affecting the development of vent pecking and cannibalism in free-range and organic laying hens. *Animal Welfare* 24, 101–111.

Lewis, P.D. and Gous, R.M. (2009) Responses of poultry to ultraviolet radiation. *World's Poultry Science Journal* 65(03), 499–510.

Lewis, P. and Morris, T. (2006) *Poultry Lighting: the Theory and Practice*. Northcot, Andover, UK.

Lisney, T.J., Rubene, D., Rozsa, J., Lovlie, H., Hastad, O. and Odeen, A. (2011) Behavioural assessment of flicker fusion frequency in chicken *Gallus gallus domesticus*. *Vision Research* 51, 1324–1332.

Marchant-Forde, R.M., Fahey, A.G. and Cheng, H.W. (2008) Comparative effects of infrared and one-third hot-blade trimming on beak topography, behavior, and growth. *Poultry Science* 87, 1474–1483.

Matkovic, K., Vucemilo, M., Vinkovic, B. and Benic, M. (2009) *Air Quality and Welfare of Cage Housed Laying Hens.* Tribun EU, Brno, Czech Republic.

Mohammed, H.H., Grashorn, M.A. and Bessei, W. (2010) The effects of lighting conditions on the behaviour of laying hens. *Archiv Fur Geflugelkunde* 74, 197–202.

Moinard, C., Statham, P., Haskell, M.J., McCorquodale, C., Jones, R.B. and Green, P.R. (2004) Accuracy of laying hens in jumping upwards and downwards between perches in different light environments. *Applied Animal Behaviour Science* 85, 77–92.

Nagle, T.A.D. and Glatz, P.C. (2012) Free range hens use the range more when the outdoor environment is enriched. *Asian-Australasian Journal of Animal Sciences* 25, 584–591.

Nicol, C.J., Bestman, M., Gilani, A.-M., De Haas, E.N., De Jong, I.C. *et al.* (2013) The prevention and control of feather pecking: application to commercial systems. *World's Poultry Science Journal* 69, 775–788.

Palczynski, L.J., Buller, H., Lambton, S.L. and Weeks, C.A. (2016) Farmer attitudes to injurious pecking in laying hens and to potential control strategies. *Animal Welfare* 25, 29–38.

Potzsch, C.J., Lewis, K., Nicol, C.J. and Green, L.E. (2001) A cross-sectional study of the prevalence of vent pecking in laying hens in alternative systems and its associations with feather pecking, management and disease. *Applied Animal Behaviour Science* 74, 259–272.

Prescott, N.B., Jarvis, J.R. and Wathes, C.M. (2004) Vision in the laying hen. In: Perry, G.C. (ed.) *Welfare of the Laying Hen*. CAB International, Wallingford, UK, pp. 155–164.

Rodenburg, T.B., Buitenhuis, A.J., Ask, B., Uitdehaag, K.A., Koene, P. *et al.* (2004a) Genetic and phenotypic correlations between feather pecking and open-field response in laying hens at two different ages. *Behavior Genetics* 34(4), 407–415.

Rodenburg, T.B., van Hierden, Y.M., Buitenhuis, A.J., Riedstra, B., Koene, P. *et al.* (2004b) Feather pecking in laying hens: new insights and directions for research? *Applied Animal Behaviour Science* 86 (3–4), 291–298.

Rodenburg, T.B., de Haas, E.N., Nielsen, B.L. and Buitenhuis, A.J. (2010) Fearfulness and feather damage in laying hens divergently selected for high and low feather pecking. *Applied Animal Behaviour Science* 128 (1–4), 91–96.

Rodenburg, T.B., De Reu, K. and Tuyttens, F.A.M. (2012) Performance, welfare, health and hygiene of laying hens in non-cage systems in comparison with cage systems. In: Sandilands, V. and Hocking, P.M. (eds) *Alternative Systems for Poultry: Health, Welfare and Productivity.* CAB International, Wallingford, UK, pp. 210–224.

Rodenburg, T.B., van Krimpen, M.M., De Jong, I.C., De Haas, E.N., Kops, M.S. *et al.* (2013) The prevention and control of feather pecking in laying hens: identifying the underlying principles. *World's Poultry Science Journal* 69, 361–374.

Savory, C.J. (1995) Feather pecking and cannibalism. *World's Poultry Science Journal* 51, 215–219.

Selvam, S., Thirunavukkarasu, M. and Kathiravan, G. (2004) Factors influencing loss due to diseases in layer farms. *Cheiron* 33, 13–17.

Thiele, H.H. and Pottguter, R. (2008) Management recommendations for laying hens in deep litter, perchery and free range systems. *Lohmann Information* 43, 53–63.

Valiente Moro, C., De Luna, C.J., Tod, A., Guy, J.H., Sparagano, O.A.E. and Zenner, L. (2009) The poultry red mite (*Dermanyssus gallinae*): a potential vector of pathogenic agents. *Experimental and Applied Acarology* 48, 93–104.

Van de Weerd, H.A. and Elson, A. (2006) Rearing factors that influence the propensity for injurious feather pecking in laying hens. *World's Poultry Science Journal* 62, 654–664.

Van Krimpen, M.M., Kwakkel, R.P., Reuvekamp, B.F.J., Van der Peet-Schwering, C.M.C., Den Hartog, L.A. and Verstegen, M.W.A. (2005) Impact of feeding management on feather pecking in laying hens. *World's Poultry Science Journal* 61, 663–685.

Van Krimpen, M.M., Kwakkel, R.P., Van der Peet-Schwering, C.M.C., Den Hartog, L.A. and Verstegen, M.W.A. (2009) Effects of nutrient dilution and nonstarch polysaccharide concentration in rearing and laying diets on eating behavior and feather damage of rearing and laying hens. *Poultry Science* 88, 759–773.

Vestergaard, K.S., Skadhauge, E. and Lawson, L.G. (1997) The stress of not being able to perform dustbathing in laying hens. *Physiology & Behavior* 62, 413–419.

Weitzenburger, D., Vits, A., Hamann, H. and Distl, O. (2005) Effect of furnished small group housing systems and furnished cages on mortality and causes of death in two layer strains. *British Poultry Science* 46, 553–559.

Widowski, T.M., Hemsworth, P.H., Barnett, J.L. and Rault, J.-L. (2016) Laying hen welfare I. Social environment and space. *World's Poultry Science Journal* 72, 333–342.

CHAPTER 6
Contact Dermatitis in Domestic Poultry

Paul M. Hocking[1*] and Teun Veldkamp[2†]

[1]Roslin Institute and R(D)SVS, University of Edinburgh, UK; [2]Wageningen Livestock Research, Wageningen, The Netherlands

ABSTRACT

Contact dermatitis is a common finding in commercial poultry kept for meat production that has both economic and welfare implications. The disease commonly affects the epidermis of the foot pad, hock joint and skin covering the breast muscles that are in contact with the litter or other floor materials. Welfare legislation in Europe has been implemented that requires farmers to reduce stocking rates if broiler chickens presented at the abattoir have a certain prevalence of foot pad dermatitis (FPD) as a proxy for poor welfare during the rearing. It has long been known that birds kept in deep litter systems are affected by foot pad dermatitis and hock burns if the litter contains too much water. The moisture content of the litter is affected by many factors (e.g. litter substrate, humidity, air temperature, stocking rate and gut health). Recently it was shown that adding water to clean wood shavings was sufficient to induce FPD and that the prevalence and severity of disease increased linearly above a certain minimum water content. The role of excess minerals, particularly sodium, and high electrolyte balance have been associated with increasing litter moisture and contact dermatitis. Hock burns and breast burns have a similar aetiology as FPD and have also been linked with high litter ammonia. Breast buttons (focal ulcerative dermatitis) and breast blisters (sternal bursitis) may be associated with poor breast feathering that exposes the naked skin to the litter. FPD, hock burns and focal ulcerative dermatitis have a similar aetiology whereas sternal bursitis is probably related to friction. FPD is associated with a cytokine milieu that is consistent with an inflammatory reaction but the precise stimulus for this response is not known with certainty. FPD has also been reported in laying hens and broiler breeders and is more prevalent in non-cage systems and in birds with outdoor access. Research

*Dr Paul Hocking passed away during the preparation of this article.
†teun.veldkamp@wur.nl

indicates that optimum dietary concentrations of vitamins and minerals are necessary to maximize skin health and that management practices must be employed to create dry, friable litter in order to minimize contact dermatitis.

INTRODUCTION

Contact dermatitis (CD) is a pathological response of skin that is in contact with the surface of the floor, whether litter, perch, slat or other hard surface. It occurs in the areas of the body that are devoid of feathers – the foot and toe pads, hock and breast. The primary disorders occur in meat birds (broilers, turkeys and ducks) and became economically significant in 2009 when the European Union (EU) legislated to control the permitted stocking density of broiler chickens in commercial farms based on the prevalence of foot pad dermatitis (FPD) in previous flocks (EU Broiler Directive, 2007/43/EC). Industry leaders assumed that similar controls would be introduced for other poultry and subsequent research in turkeys to reduce FPD was initiated. Furthermore, with the opening of the Chinese market, an outlet for chicken feet was created that necessitates clean feet unaffected by FPD.

There are five types of contact dermatitis occurring in meat poultry: foot and toe pad dermatitis (which will be lumped together as FPD), breast blisters (sternal bursitis, SB), breast buttons (focal ulcerative dermatitis, FUD), breast burns (BB) and hock burns (HB). Poor feathering in the breast region in modern strains of turkeys and broiler chickens exposes the skin of the breast to surface moisture, pressure and friction, resulting in BB, FUD and SB.

FPD must not be confused with bumble foot or gout. Bumble foot (ulcerative pododermatitis) is the result of a bacterial infection, usually by *Staphylococcus aureus*; it will present as a rapid onset of swelling that is hot to the touch and affected birds are clearly in pain. FPD, by comparison, is cold to touch, slow to develop, and signs of pain are not obvious. Gout occurs as a result of kidney failure or high crude protein diets, is very painful and is associated with the deposition of white uric acid crystals in the synovial capsules and tendon of the foot pad. Importantly, FPD is not accompanied by the presence of bacteria and is a physiological response to environmental irritant, chiefly high concentrations of water in the litter, the evidence for which will be presented below.

FPD has been reported in laying hens (Wang *et al.*, 1998) and broiler breeders (Kaukonen *et al.*, 2016) and is more prevalent in non-cage systems and in birds with outdoor access. There is little published information on these production systems and they will not be discussed further. This chapter will therefore summarize the measurement and prevalence of the different types of contact dermatitis and methods to reduce their prevalence in commercial flocks of meat poultry, primarily in broiler chickens and turkeys. Practical methods for managing contact dermatitis – principally husbandry practices and nutritional standards – will be outlined. A brief account of the aetiology and pathology of contact dermatitis will be presented and the economic and welfare implications of contact dermatitis will be discussed.

MEASURING CONTACT DERMATITIS

Contact dermatitis has generally been assessed using a scoring system at the slaughterhouse. Common scoring systems range from a simple binary (affected, not affected) scale to one that assesses the area of the affected skin (Hocking *et al.*, 2008). The third type of scoring system evaluates both the extent and depth or severity of the lesion (Allain *et al.*, 2009). The EU regulatory system for broiler carcasses is based on a three-point system: unaffected; mild or moderate; and severe. Each score is weighted differentially (0.0, 0.5 and 2.0, respectively) and summed over a sample of feet to give an overall flock score. Several consecutive flocks are evaluated and the mean flock scores are used to determine the stocking density that will be permitted in subsequent flocks.

Visual scoring is widely used in welfare assessment of commercial flocks in the field and on the slaughter line. A training tool for individual assessors is available for use on laptops, tablets and mobile phones that also reports repeatability and consistency among scorers to the administrator of the software (Roslin Institute and Royal (Dick) School of Veterinary Studies, Edinburgh, available at http://footpad.roslin.ed.ac.uk/footpad/). A repeatability of over 0.95 should be achieved by regular scorers and represents a practical target during training.

Recently, instruments to assess FPD in the abattoir have been introduced that automatically determine the FPD score based on the proportion of the area of the foot pad that is affected. Measurement of the surface temperature or the dialectical constant of the foot pad have been proposed as methods for assessing FPD on the slaughter line but do not appear to have been successful in early trials (Hoffmann *et al.*, 2013). Automatic machine-based methods have the potential advantage of ease of use, objectivity and comprehensiveness compared with human scorers and their use is likely to increase in future. Recent research has shown that optical flow measurement of broiler activity in commercial flocks can be used to predict the prevalence of FPD in live birds and facilitate pre-emptive husbandry changes to minimize the prevalence at slaughter (Dawkins *et al.*, 2017).

For small-scale experimental research, a finer scoring system may be adopted to aid discrimination between treatments. For example, Mayne *et al.* (2007a) used a 7-point system for external scoring (Table 6.1): the low scores on this system describe degrees of inflammation that were observable in the author's experimental system, but which are virtually impossible to detect in experiments that simulate commercial conditions. A 7-point scoring system for assessing the severity of histopathology (Table 6.2) was also described by Mayne *et al.* (2006) and this system may be adopted for both experimental and commercial samples.

PREVALENCE OF CONTACT DERMATITIS IN COMMERCIAL POULTRY FLOCKS

Many factors affect the prevalence of contact dermatitis in commercial flocks and there are relatively few publications on the prevalence in national flocks or even

Table 6.1. External foot pad scoring system (Mayne *et al.*, 2007a).

Score	Description of foot pad
0	No external signs of FPD. Skin of the foot pad and digital pads appears normal, no redness, swelling or necrosis is evident. The skin of the foot pad feels soft to the touch.
1	Slight swelling and/or redness of the skin of the foot pad.
2	The pad feels harder and denser than a non-affected foot. The central part of the pad is raised with swelling and redness and the reticulate scales may be separated. The digital pads may show a similar reaction.
3	The central and digital foot pads are enlarged and swollen with red areas, and as the skin has become compacted, the foot pad skin is harder. The reticulate scales have enlarged and separated, and small black necrotic areas may occur.
4	Marked swelling and redness around the margins of lesions occur. Reticulate scales die and turn black, forming scale-shaped necrotic areas. The scales around the outside of the black areas may have turned white. The area of necrosis is less than one-eighth of the total area of the foot pad.
5	Swelling and redness are evident in the central and digital foot pads. The total foot pad size is enlarged. Reticulate scales are pronounced, increased in number and separated from each other. The amount of necrosis extends to one-quarter of the foot pad. Small necrotic areas may also appear on the digital pads.
6	As Score 5, but with half the foot pad covered by necrotic cells. The digital pads may have up to half of one pad covered with necrotic cells.
7	A foot pad with over half of the foot pad covered in necrotic scales.

Table 6.2. Scoring system for histopathological observations of footpads (Mayne *et al.*, 2006).

Score	Description	Definition
0	None	No change, sample normal.
1	Mild	Hyperkeratosis; 'horned pegs' of keratin on surface; epithelial hyperplasia; compressed keratin on footpad surface.
2	Mild	Epidermal acanthosis; increased dermal blood vessel density.
3	Mild	Vacuoles in dermis/epidermis; necrotic debris in keratin/epidermis.
4	Medium	Presence of heterophils, macrophages and lymphocytes in dermis.
5	Medium–severe	Increased density of heterophils, macrophages and lymphocytes; congested/necrotic blood vessels; necrotic debris of cells in dermis/epidermis.
6	Severe	Split epidermis – 1 lesion.
7	Severe	Split epidermis – 1+ lesion or 1 very large lesion, more than one-third of total sample.

in a commercial enterprise, although many firms record such information. The range of FPD in a standard production system can be very wide: Haslam *et al.* (2007) reported a range of 0.0–71.5% in commercial broiler flocks in 149 farms, for example. Furthermore, Pagazaurtundua and Warriss (2006) reported a prevalence of FPD ranging from 9.6% to 98.1% in different production systems in the UK, suggesting that an overall prevalence is misleading. Nevertheless, typical results for turkey and broiler flocks in commercial intensive production systems are presented in Table 6.3 for FPD and Table 6.4 for HB, SB and FUD, respectively, to illustrate the likely prevalence in Europe.

In general, the prevalence of FPD and FUD in turkeys is greater than in broilers, probably because the turkeys are slaughtered at a greater age than broilers, allowing more time for contact with wet litter, whereas HB is more prevalent in broilers than in turkeys. St-Hilaire *et al.* (2003) reported a prevalence for SB and FUD, respectively, of 8.8% and 22.6% in over 11,700 slaughtered turkeys from 24 Canadian farms. These authors reported a positive correlation of 0.5 between these two disorders that is typical of other studies of FPD, HB and BB reflecting the importance of a single causative factor: wet litter. There is little published information on ducks but it is known that FPD is clinically significant in ducklings. Jones and Dawkins (2010) reported a prevalence of moderate and severe FPD of 13% in 46 commercial flocks of Pekin ducks.

FACTORS AFFECTING THE PREVALENCE OF FPD

The classic papers of Martland (1984, 1985) and Greene *et al.* (1985) showed that the prevalence of FPD was strongly linked to wet, sticky or caked litter. Foot pad lesions are sometimes referred to as ammonia burns but several studies have shown that litter moisture alone can cause or induce FPD (Table 6.5). Mayne *et al.* (2007a) developed an experimental system for generating FPD lesion based on a low stocking density, regular removal of excreta and soiled litter and the application of tap water to model the induction of FPD. These workers showed that FPD developed rapidly in turkeys and lesions healed after 2 weeks when re-housed on to dry, clean litter (Fig. 6.1). Using the same experimental model, the same authors showed that turkeys were susceptible from 7 to 10

Table 6.3. Typical reports of the prevalence of FPD in commercial turkey and broiler flocks.

Species	Gender	Number	Age (days)	Affected (%)	Reference
Turkeys	Male	110,000	146	90	Mayne (2006)
	Female	55,500	118	80	
	Male	11,429	–	100	Allain *et al.* (2013)
Broilers	Mixed	17,000	41	71	Allain *et al.* (2009)

Table 6.4. Comparative prevalence of hock burn, sternal bursitis and focal ulcerative dermatitis in turkeys and broiler chickens in France.

Lesion	Turkeys[a]	Broilers[b]
Hock burn (%)	4.4	59.0
Sternal bursitis (%)	1.5	4.2
Focal ulcerative dermatitis (%)	31.0	15.8

[a]Allain *et al.* (2013); [b]Allain *et al.* (2009).

weeks of age. Weber Wyneken *et al.* (2015) showed that increasing the water content of the litter above a certain proportion resulted in a linear increase in the mean FPD score. These experiments, using clean litter and added water, clearly demonstrated that water alone was sufficient to induce FPD. Experimental evidence from human and animal studies support this conclusion (see below). The presence of ammonia or other chemical substances such as uric acid in the litter may play a role in the further development of FPD but does not appear to be a primary cause. Similarly, common intestinal diseases have been linked to FPD through an effect on litter moisture (e.g. coccidiosis, *Clostridium perfringens* and *Escherichia coli*).

Environmental factors affect litter moisture content and have been extensively reviewed elsewhere (Mayne, 2005). These include management and

Table 6.5. The effects of 6 days of high litter moisture in clean wood shavings on the prevalence of foot pad dermatitis in turkeys (Mayne *et al.*, 2007a). External and histopathology slides were scored on 7-point scales.

		Mean score, day 6	
Litter	Moisture (%)	External	Histopathology
Dry, clean	13	0.7	2.5
Wet, clean	74	6.3	6.5
SED	2.2***	0.53***	0.41***

***$P < 0.001$

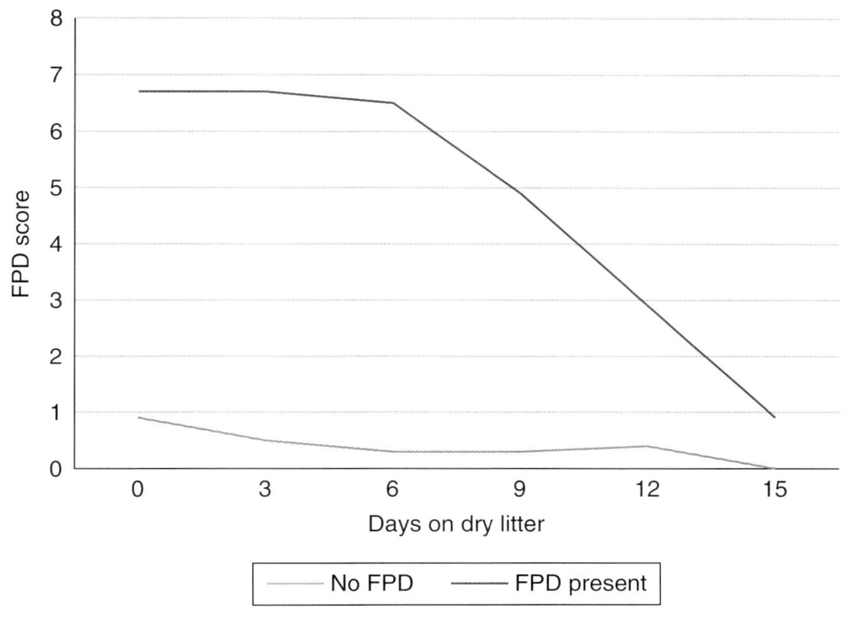

Fig. 6.1. Mean footpad scores at 3-day intervals after housing 23-day-old turkeys on dry litter following 48 h on wet or dry litter (Mayne *et al.*, 2007a).

housing (type of litter, litter depth, distribution of light, light colour, photoperiod, ambient temperature, ventilation, relative humidity, drinking system, stocking density) and dietary factors that affect water consumption and excreta composition and the capacity of the litter to retain moisture and limit evaporative water loss. In addition, specific nutrient deficiencies, particularly of zinc and biotin, may affect the ability of the epidermis to resist an environmental insult. Finally, susceptibility to CD is also influenced by genetic factors, which are discussed in Chapter 10 of this volume. For up-to-date information on environmental management the reader should refer to the current management manuals published by the breeding companies. Good husbandry and disease control are the primary mechanisms for decreasing the prevalence of CD in commercial flocks.

Much of the research on CD has focused on FPD and HB and it will be assumed that both are primarily the result of wet litter. There is little information on the causes of FUD, which may be the result of a localized infection of a feather follicle whereas SB is probably caused by friction associated with regular transitions from resting to standing and may be exacerbated in birds with relatively heavy breast muscles. The relative lack of feather cover in commercial broilers and turkeys undoubtedly contributes to the likelihood of developing breast lesions: Miner and Smart (1975) covered the breast with sheepskin in range-reared turkeys and this led to a significant reduction in the prevalence of breast blisters.

AETIOLOGY AND PATHOLOGY OF CONTACT DERMATITIS

The epidermis serves to protect the body from the environment and is composed of differentiating keratinocytes. Little recent avian research has been conducted into the structure and functions of avian skin, in contrast to the large body of literature for the human and murine skin. These species are, of course, adapted to a terrestrial environment and it will be assumed here that relevant research in these species is broadly relevant to poultry.

The final cornified layer of cells – corneocytes – are directly exposed to the litter, perch or soil and vegetation. Corneocytes are anucleated cells that are biologically dead but serve as an essential physical, chemical and immunological barrier. The major intracellular keratin filaments form filaggrins (filament aggregating proteins) that provide structural integrity to the cell and a scaffold for the extracellular lipid matrix (Elias, 2007; Kezic and Jakasa, 2016). When filaggrin is degraded, the resulting small molecules and natural moisturizing factors account, in part, for the acidic pH and water-holding capacity of skin (Kezic and Jakasa, 2016). When there is excess moisture in the litter, the epidermis is eroded and the deep layers of the skin are exposed to a physiological insult that elicits an immune cytokine response (Mayne *et al.*, 2007c). The hypothesis that water per se is sufficient to cause FPD and similar conditions finds support from experiments with laboratory animals, swine and human skin exposed to pure water for several hours, in which the response is similar in terms of both time course and pathology to that observed in FPD (Jolly and Swan, 1980; Kligman, 1994; Ramsing and Agner, 1997; Warner *et al.*, 1999). Whereas compounds in the litter such as ammonia (Sherlock *et al.*, 2012), excreta (e.g. uric acid) or litter material (e.g. phenols and resins in softwood shavings) (Ayars *et al.*, 1989) may exacerbate the response following exposure to high litter moisture, it is likely that this is a secondary effect to the role of water in causing FPD, HB and BB.

ROLE OF NUTRITION ON LITTER QUALITY AND THE PREVALENCE OF CONTACT DERMATITIS

Dietary factors affecting litter moisture, usually with particular reference to FPD, have been extensively researched (Mayne, 2005). In recent years several papers have described the effects of high dietary crude protein concentrations, the use of soybean meal as the main or even sole source of protein and the effects of a high electrolyte balance on litter moisture and/or FPD. Excessive dietary protein supply in birds must be catabolized and excreted via the kidneys in the form of uric acid – which implies higher water consumption – and secondary production of ammonia. Soybean meal, the main protein source in poultry diets, contains other components that can be responsible for a higher water excretion, such as fibre with high water-retention capacity, fermentable sugars and potassium. Recently, Veldkamp *et al.* (2017) and Hocking *et al.* (2018) studied the effect of feed ingredients on litter moisture and FPD in turkeys. Veldkamp *et al.* (2017) studied the effect of crude protein concentration and dietary electrolyte balance on litter quality, FPD, growth performance and processing yields in two medium-heavy turkey hybrids. Soybean meal was replaced by vegetable protein sources selected for lower potassium concentrations to lower dietary electrolyte balance (DEB) in order to improve litter quality and subsequent quality of foot pads. The effects of crude protein (CP) on litter friability and wetness were not consistent during the production period. FPD in turkeys fed on diets with low CP was significantly lower than FPD in turkeys fed on diets with high CP until 84 days. Litter was significantly drier in pens of turkeys fed on diets with low DEB than in pens of turkeys fed on diets with high DEB. FPD in turkeys fed on diets with low DEB was significantly lower than in turkeys fed on diets with high DEB. Growth performance and processing yields were adversely affected at low DEB. From this study it was concluded that litter quality can be improved and FPD may be decreased in turkeys fed on diets containing lower CP and DEB levels. Hocking *et al.* (2018) observed that soybean meal increases litter moisture and FPD in maize- and wheat-based diets for turkeys. A 2×2 factorial experiment was conducted to compare the effects of wheat- or maize-based diets differing in DEB on litter moisture and FPD at 4, 8 and 12 weeks of age in heavy-medium turkeys. A second objective was to investigate the effects on FPD of the interaction between dietary composition and artificially increasing litter moisture by adding water to the litter. High DEB diets contained soybean as the main protein source whereas low DEB diets did not contain soybean meal. Litter moisture and mean FPD score were higher in turkeys fed on high DEB diets compared with low DEB diets. Hocking *et al.* (2018) also concluded that lowering DEB for turkeys may improve litter moisture and lower the prevalence of FPD in commercial turkey flocks. Similarly, in broilers, the effects of nutrition on prevalence and severity of

FPD have been studied. For example, Van Harn and Veldkamp (2005) studied reducing CP levels in broiler diets on a daily basis by adding whole wheat. These authors showed that whole-wheat feeding resulted in a better litter quality and less severe FPD. Body weight gain and feed conversion ratio were decreased compared with the control. The CP intake of the whole-wheat-fed broilers was 13% lower compared with the control group.

The provision of sodium, potassium or phosphorus but not calcium in concentrations above established recommendations results in a linear increase in water intake (Smith *et al.*, 2000). Vitamins such as zinc and biotin are essential for the development of skin integrity. Dietary provision for biotin greatly in excess of commercial recommendations for turkeys was suggested to decrease FPD but the claim was not confirmed in a controlled experiment (Mayne *et al.*, 2007b). These examples emphasize the role of the nutritionist in managing wet litter and avoiding excessive dietary costs.

MANAGEMENT FACTORS TO REDUCE THE PREVALENCE OF CONTACT DERMATITIS

In turkeys, Vinco *et al.* (2018) studied the effects of different management factors on FPD in turkeys. Company vertical integration was one of the most influential factors, most probably due to the role of feed composition which was confounded with integration. Drinker type, drinker number and litter type were the main factors affecting litter moisture and FPD. Litter moisture was confirmed to be correlated to the incidence of FPD in these commercial flocks. Litter moisture, measured by visual monitoring and scoring, appeared to be more reliable in predicting the prevalence of FPD than laboratory or objective methods such as measuring the dry matter content in the litter.

In broilers, many studies on the effects of management factors on FPD have been conducted. As an example, the effects of litter material, litter thickness, drinker types and lighting regimes are reported here. In Northern European countries, wood shavings and chopped wheat straw (to increase water absorption capacity) are the most commonly used litter materials for broilers. Currently other materials such as peat, lignocellulose, rapeseed straw and maize silage are also being used as litter material in broiler houses. Litter material does affect FPD. German research found that, compared with wood shavings and chopped straw, the use of lignocellulose (Pelletino® Strohstreugranulat G) reduced FPD (Berk, 2009). De Baere and Zoons (2004) compared chopped wheat straw and wood shavings as litter material for broilers. Broiler performance did not differ between the two litter materials, but less FPD was found to occur on wood shavings. In general, the more absorbent the litter material, the lower was the incidence of FPD. The use of peat as a litter material for broilers reduced the severity of FPD (Bilgili *et al.*, 2009; Kaukonen *et al.*, 2017). In general, nipple drinkers reduce water spillage compared with drinking systems with drinking cups; this decreases the risk of wet litter and FPD (Ekstrand *et al.*, 1997). Light has also been shown to affect FPD: studies in The Netherlands and Belgium have shown that intermittent light schedules decrease the occurrence of FPD (de Baere, 2008; Van Harn, 2009). In managing litter conditions to minimize CD, regular replacement of very wet or caked litter with fresh material is essential, particularly in broiler and duck flocks that are slaughtered at a relatively young age. Some commercial flock owners have resorted to underfloor heating to maintain dry litter conditions in broiler flocks and was shown to be effective in a turkey experiment (Abd El-Wahab *et al.*, 2011). Regular turning of litter in turkey flocks, which are housed for a relatively long period, using a garden rotavator will assist in the maintenance of good litter conditions by mixing the spoiled surface litter with the relatively dry subsurface litter.

Recent technical developments may assist the day-to-day management of litter conditions: robots have been developed to turn over the litter on a daily basis and these, with the development of suitable sensors, could be used to alert the flock manager when any of the environmental conditions warranted human management input. This particular innovation has the benefit of assessing the environment at the level at which the bird experiences it.

ECONOMIC AND WELFARE IMPLICATIONS OF CONTACT DERMATITIS

Controlling the water content of poultry litter to minimize CD, specifically FPD and HB, inevitably increases the cost of production. Higher ventilation rates, heating, more expensive litter (e.g. wood shavings versus chopped straw), labour for turning over the litter and removal of soiled litter will all add to the cost of production. However, profitability is not necessarily affected, as there is evidence in commercial broiler flocks and the experiments with turkeys that, for example, wet litter and high FPD score are associated with lower productivity (De Jong *et al.*, 2014).

Short-term experiments with growing turkeys showed slower growth rates or increased food intakes in birds on very wet litter (Mayne *et al.*, 2007a). It is likely that both broilers and turkeys on wet litter lose heat more rapidly to the environments as water evaporates from their almost featherless breast skin.

Turkeys housed on wet litter show greatly reduced levels of activity, indicative of pain or discomfort (Wu and Hocking, 2011). Furthermore, when turkeys with FPD associated with wet litter were re-housed on dry litter, activity immediately increased but did not reach the level in turkeys housed on dry litter with no FPD (Sinclair *et al.*, 2015). These results suggest that turkeys with FPD housed on wet litter experience a decrease in affective state in addition to potential pain associated with FPD and HB.

Weber Wynken *et al.* (2015) used gait analysis in two medium heavy turkey strains to assess the painfulness of FPD independently of litter condition. The birds were allowed to walk over a pressure platform to measure gait parameters in birds with or without FPD given analgesia (betamethasone) or saline injections. Turkeys with high FPD scores were slower than those with low FPD scores and had greater double support time, lower stride length and stance time, consistent with slower walking speed. However, the intervention of analgesia and FPD score was not significant and gait parameters were similar for birds given saline or betamethasone. It is difficult, therefore, to conclude from these results that FPD causes pain.

Sinclair *et al.* (2015) studied house pen behaviour. Turkeys were housed on wet or dry litter for 17 days and given daily injections of betamethasone from day 10 to day 17. Video recordings of house pen behaviour were conducted on day 15 and at 1500 h on day 16. Birds on wet litter (FPD score 6.3) were transferred to the dry litter pens and birds on dry litter (FPD score 0.5) to pens with wet litter. Video recordings were then conducted on day 17.

Statistically significant interactions between FPD score, analgesia and litter condition occurred for the percentage of time resting and standing. High-FPD birds transferred to wet litter given betamethasone rested less than those given saline; a similar difference occurred between high-FPD birds on wet litter, but the differences on dry litter were small. Similar changes, with sign reversed, occurred for the percentage of time standing.

A second analysis of the data that measured unique patterns of behaviour (variety, frequency and complexity) was conducted under the premise that FPD pain would disrupt regular behavioural sequences. Statistically significant interactions between FPD score and wet or dry litter were observed. Low-FPD birds had a similar pattern of behaviour on both wet and dry litter. Whereas behavioural sequences of high-FPD birds transferred from wet to dry litter increased, the number of unique sequences was still less than in high-FPD birds housed on dry litter. There were no interactions involving FPD score, litter and analgesia. It was concluded that wet litter, per se, resulted in poor welfare, but that attentional biases and affective states were likely to affect pain perception.

CONCLUSIONS

There are two incentives to reduce the incidence of FPD by controlling litter moisture: (i) it may be economically more profitable to do so; and (ii) the overall welfare of the birds is compromised on wet litter. Furthermore, in broiler chickens in Europe there is the added incentive of legislative and economic pressure to do so. Whether pain is associated with FPD, or any of the other forms of CD, is currently not proven, but it would be remarkable if they were not painful, depending on the severity of the lesion.

REFERENCES

Abd El-Wahab, A., Beineke, A., Beyerbach, M., Visscher, C.F. and Kamphues, J. (2011) Effects of floor heating and litter quality on the development and severity of foot pad dermatitis in young turkeys. *Avian Diseases* 55, 429–434.

Allain, V., Mirabito, L., Arnould, C., Colas, M., Le Bouquin, S., Lupo, C. and Michel, V. (2009) Skin lesions in broiler chickens measured at the slaughterhouse: relationships between lesions and between their prevalence and rearing factors. *British Poultry Science* 50, 407–417.

Allain, V., Huonnic, D., Rouina, M. and Michel, V. (2013) Prevalence of skin lesions in turkeys at slaughter. *British Poultry Science* 54, 33–41.

Ayars, G.H., Altman, L.C., Frazier, C.E. and Chi, E.Y. (1989) The toxicity of constituents of cedar and pine woods to pulmonary epithelium. *Journal of Allergy and Clinical Immunology* 83, 610–618.

Berk, J. (2009) Effect of litter type on prevalence and severity of pododermatitis in male broilers. *Berliner Und Munchener Tierarztliche Wochenschrift* 122, 257–263.

Bilgili, S.F., Hess, J.B., Blake, J.P., Macklin, K.S., Saenmahayak, B. and Sibley, J.L. (2009) Influence of bedding material on footpad dermatitis in broiler chickens. *Journal of Applied Poultry Research* 18, 583–589.

Dawkins, M.S., Roberts, S.J., Cain, R.J., Nickson, T. and Donnelly, C.A. (2017) Early warning of footpad dermatitis and hockburn in broiler chicken flocks using optical flow, bodyweight and water consumption. *Veterinary Record* 180, 499–499.

de Baere, K. (2008) Lichtschema's bij vleeskuikens. *Pluimvee* 46 [in Dutch].

de Baere, K. and Zoons, J. (2004) Strooiselmateriaal in pluimveestallen. *Pluimvee* 40 [in Dutch].

De Jong, I.C., Gunnink, H. and Van Harn, J. (2014) Wet litter not only induces footpad dermatitis but also reduces overall welfare, technical performance, and carcass yield in broiler chickens. *Journal of Applied Poultry Research* 23(1), 51–58.

Ekstrand, C., Algers, B. and Svedberg, J. (1997) Rearing conditions and foot-pad dermatitis in Swedish broiler chickens. *Preventive Veterinary Medicine* 31, 167–174.

Elias, P.M. (2007) The skin barrier as an innate immune element. *Seminars in Immunopathology* 29, 3.

Greene, J.A., McCracken, R.M. and Evans, R.T. (1985) A contact-dermatitis of broilers – clinical and pathological findings. *Avian Pathology* 14(1), 23–38.

Haslam, S.M., Knowles, T.G., Brown, S.N., Wilkins, L.J., Kestin, S.C., Warriss, P.D. and Nicol, C.J. (2007) Factors affecting the prevalence of foot pad dermatitis, hock burn and breast burn in broiler chicken. *British Poultry Science* 48, 264–275.

Hocking, P.M., Mayne, R.K., Else, R.W., French, N.A. and Gatcliffe, J. (2008) Standard European footpad dermatitis scoring system for use in turkey processing plants. *World's Poultry Science Journal* 64(03), 323–328.

Hocking, P.M., Vinco, L.J. and Veldkamp, T. (2018) Soya bean meal increases litter moisture and foot pad dermatitis in maize and wheat based diets for turkeys but maize and non-soya diets lower body weight. *British Poultry Science* 59(2), 227–231.

Hoffmann, G., Ammon, C., Volkamer, L., Suerie, C. and Radko, D. (2013) Sensor-based monitoring of the prevalence and severity of foot pad dermatitis in broiler chickens. *British Poultry Science* 54, 553–561.

Jolly, M. and Swan, A.G. (1980) The effects on rat skin of prolonged exposure to water. *British Journal of Dermatology* 103, 387–395.

Jones, T.A. and Dawkins, M.S. (2010) Environment and management factors affecting Pekin duck production and welfare on commercial farms in the UK. *British Poultry Science* 51, 12–21.

Kaukonen, E., Norring, M. and Valros, A. (2016) Effect of litter quality on foot pad dermatitis, hock burns and breast blisters in broiler breeders during the production period. *Avian Pathology* 45, 667–673.

Kaukonen, E., Norring, M. and Valros, A. (2017) Evaluating the effects of bedding materials and elevated platforms on contact dermatitis and plumage cleanliness of commercial broilers and on litter condition in broiler houses. *British Poultry Science* 58, 480–489.

Kezic, S. and Jakasa, I. (2016) Filaggrin and skin barrier function. In: Agner, T. (ed.) *Skin Barrier Function*, Vol. 49. Karger, Basel, pp. 1–7.

Kligman, A.M. (1994) Hydration injury to human skin. In: Elsner, P., Berardesca, E. and Maibach, H.I. (eds) *Bioengineering of the Skin: Water and the Stratum Corneum*. CRC Press, Boca Raton, Florida, pp. 251–255.

Martland, M.F. (1984) Wet litter as a cause of plantar pododermatitis leading to foot ulceration and lameness in fattening turkeys. *Avian Pathology* 13, 241–252.

Martland, M.F. (1985) Ulcerative dermatitis in broiler chickens: the effects of wet litter. *Avian Pathology* 14, 353–364.

Mayne, R.K. (2005) A review of the aetiology and possible causative factors of foot pad dermatitis in growing turkeys and broilers. *World's Poultry Science Journal* 61, 256–267.

Mayne, R.K. (2006) Decreasing the prevalence of foot pad dermatitits in commercial turkeys. University of Edinburgh.

Mayne, R.K., Hocking, P.M. and Else, R.W. (2006) Foot pad dermatitis develops at an early age in commercial turkeys. *British Poultry Science* 47, 36–42.

Mayne, R.K., Else, R.W. and Hocking, P.M. (2007a) High litter moisture alone is sufficient to cause footpad dermatitis in growing turkeys. *British Poultry Science* 48, 538–545.

Mayne, R.K., Else, R.W. and Hocking, P.M. (2007b) High dietary concentrations of biotin did not prevent foot pad dermatitis in growing turkeys and external scores were poor indicators of histopathological lesions. *British Poultry Science* 48, 291–298.

Mayne, R.K., Powell, F., Else, R.W., Kaiser, P. and Hocking, P.M. (2007c) Foot pad dermatitis in growing turkeys is associated with cytokine and cellular changes indicative of an inflammatory immune response. *Avian Pathology* 36, 453–459.

Miner, M.L. and Smart, R.A. (1975) Causes of enlarged sternal bursas (breast blisters). *Avian Diseases* 19, 246–256.

Pagazaurtundua, A. and Warriss, P.D. (2006) Levels of foot pad dermatitis in broiler chickens reared in 5 different systems. *British Poultry Science* 47, 529–532.

Ramsing, D.W. and Agner, T. (1997) Effect of water on experimentally irritated human skin. *British Journal of Dermatology* 136, 364–367.

Sherlock, L., McKeegan, D.E.F., Cheng, Z., Wathes, C.M. and Wathes, D.C. (2012) Effects of contact dermatitis on hepatic gene expression in broilers. *British Poultry Science* 53, 439–452.

Sinclair, A C., Wyneken, W., Veldkamp, T., Vinco, L.J. and Hocking, P.M. (2015) Behavioural assessment of pain in commercial turkeys (*Meleagris gallopavo*) with foot pad dermatitis. *British Poultry Science* 56(5), 511–521.

Smith, A., Rose, S.P., Wells, R.G. and Pirgozliev, V. (2000) Effect of excess dietary sodium, potassium, calcium and phosphorus on excreta moisture of laying hens. *British Poultry Science* 41, 598–607.

St-Hilaire, S., Arellano, S. and Ribble, C. (2003) Association between cellulitis (enlarged sternal bursa) and focal ulcerative dermatitis in ontario turkeys at the time of processing. *Avian Diseases* 47, 531–536.

Van Harn, J. (2009) Invulling lichteisen EU-welzijnsrichtlijn voor vleeskuikens – vier lichtschema's vergeleken. *ASG-Rapport* 172 [in Dutch].

Van Harn, J. and Veldkamp, T. (2005) Dynamisch voeren belooft veel goed, maar . . . er valt nog wat te sleutelen! *De Pluimveehouderij* 35(8), 14–15 [in Dutch].

Veldkamp, T., Hocking, P.M. and Vinco, L.J. (2017) Effect of crude protein concentration and dietary electrolyte balance on litter quality, foot pad dermatitis, growth performance and processing yields in two medium heavy turkey hybrids. *British Poultry Science* 58, 557–568.

Vinco, L.J., Giacomelli, S., Campana, L., Chiari, M., Vitale, N. *et al.* (2018) Identification of a practical and reliable method for the evaluation of litter moisture in turkey production. *British Poultry Science* 59, 7–12.

Wang, G., Ekstrand, C. and Svedberg, J. (1998) Wet litter and perches as risk factors for the development of foot pad dermatitis in floor-housed hens. *British Poultry Science* 39, 191–197.

Warner, R.R., Boissy, Y.L., Lilly, N.A., Spears, M.J., McKillop, K., Marshall, J.L. and Stone, K.J. (1999) Water disrupts stratum corneum lipid lamellae: damage is similar to surfactants. *Journal of Investigative Dermatology* 113, 960–966.

Weber Wyneken, C., Sinclair, A., Veldkamp, T., Vinco, L.J. and Hocking, P.M. (2015) Footpad dermatitis and pain assessment in turkey poults using analgesia and objective gait analysis. *British Poultry Science* 56, 522–530.

Wu, K. and Hocking, P.M. (2011) Turkeys are equally susceptible to foot pad dermatitis from 1 to 10 weeks of age and foot pad scores were minimized when litter moisture was less than 30%. *Poultry Science* 90, 1170–1178.

CHAPTER 7
The Poultry Integument in Health and Disease

Paul F. McMullin*

Poultry Health International, Thirsk, North Yorkshire, UK

ABSTRACT

The importance of the integumentary system in commercial poultry encompasses all its functions that are essential to maintaining the health of the bird. Much can be learned about the health condition of the birds in a flock by observation of presence, or absence, and distribution of feathers on the floor in the house, as well as from plumage quality, feather loss and skin condition.

Development and colouration of wattles and combs can also be a useful guide to flock health and physiological status. Patterns of skin damage, where present, and plumage loss allow inference of bird behaviour. Close inspection of growing feathers can also provide indications of both physiological and infectious issues during the time that feathers were being formed. The integumentary system of poultry can provide useful information to help to improve management and monitor and control specific diseases, thereby maintaining and improving health, welfare and productivity of farmed poultry. In this chapter, various issues associated with the skin, feather and beak as well as during slaughter process are discussed.

INTRODUCTION

The integumentary system of birds encompasses both body skin and that of specialized organs such as chicken comb and wattles, as well as the appendages, the feathers of various sorts, beak horn, toe nails and scales, and is the most varied of any vertebrate class. The importance of the integumentary system to health in commercial poultry includes all of the functions associated with the integument in other species, such as maintenance of underlying tissue moisture,

*paulmcmullin@poultryhealthinternational.net

temperature regulation, protection of internal organs, prevention of microbial invasion and synthesis of vitamin D. There is a broad range of disease conditions affecting these structures and space does not permit coverage of all of these here. For those with a particular interest in this area, and in particular the pathology, there is an excellent review available (Pass, 1989). This chapter will provide some updates on developments in this area over the past 30 years, from the perspective of a specialist poultry veterinarian.

CLINICAL INSPECTION

For the poultry farmer and practising veterinarian, the appearance of visible areas of skin and associated structures is very useful in assessing flock health. Plumage development and persistence can be indicative of nutritional status, behaviour and management. Careful observations made of the patterns of skin damage, where present, and plumage loss can be a useful guide to bird behaviour. Close inspection of growing feathers can also provide indications of both physiological and systemic infectious issues during the time that feather was being formed. Even the presence, type and amount of shed feathers on the floor is informative, given that it is normal for a degree of feather loss to occur through life. If the shed feathers 'disappear' this usually indicates that they are being consumed, which can be a precursor to progressive feather pecking and, eventually, cannibalism. Development and colour of comb, wattles and exposed skin on the legs are indicative of sexual development in the chicken. These observations contribute to a general assessment of flock health, as well as allowing us to focus on individuals that merit more detailed examination. In housed poultry the presence and distribution of dust, partly derived from skin and feathers, also helps us to understand aspects of ventilation.

ISSUES AND DISEASES ASSOCIATED WITH THE SKIN

Trauma

Much of the trauma that occurs is due to interaction with flock-mates, as a result of either pecking or toe-claw injuries. Most minor scratches and abrasions heal well and are of limited health and welfare consequence. However, good managers pay attention to any damage as it can act as a trigger for cannibalism or entry of secondary local, or systemic, infections. Other forms of trauma include physical (litter with sharp splinters, or larger pieces of wood) and chemical (as a result of wet litter with resultant contact dermatitis). Caked litter with resultant 'sharp edges' is associated with 'breast blisters' (synovitis of the sternal bursa) in meat turkeys. Avoidance of damage to the skin and mucosa at the margin of the vent is particularly important, as it can have significant systemic effects. In addition to loss of normal cloacal function and consequent leaking of urate solution, damaged vents in females can result in blood staining of egg shells and interrupt the normal cycle of oviposition, contributing to the subsequent development of peritonitis. Cloacitis in turkey parents has been associated with transfer of mature birds on to litter with fine particles of disintegrated wood bedding. Vent damage in laying chickens is typically seen on the ventral margin of the vent and progresses to bands of dry gangrene. While the exact cause of this is currently unknown, it may be hypothesized that it is the result of a mismatch between egg size and cloacal development, or mild vent pecking in communal nest boxes. Minimizing the use of nest-box lights (which are commonly used in early lay to attract birds into the boxes) does appear to be helpful in reducing vent damage and improving liveability.

Much of the skin damage encountered is a result of bird-to-bird interaction but it can be significantly affected by genetics, bird management and the other disease factors discussed here. In meat-type breeding chickens, careful management of feeding and weights is critically important in avoiding wounds. In all breeding poultry with natural mating, compliance with breed recommendations for bird weights and mating ratios helps to reduce the risk of injury and improve production. If a disease condition affects the females preferentially, it is important to reduce the number of males in proportion to the female losses to avoid damage related to over-mating. Maintenance of an appropriate and even light intensity is usually helpful in avoiding pecking, feather plucking and similar issues. This is important over the whole floor area and also over time. Shafts of sunlight reaching a bird can attract other birds to peck at the area illuminated, even if it is another bird. Where controlled-lighting housing is in use it is particularly important to ensure that light entry at a time of day when the house lights are off does not result in activity of part of the flock. The equipment should be designed to allow birds to perch safely and not be subject to feather plucking by birds passing underneath them.

Fungi and ectoparasites

Fungal infections and most types of ectoparasites are usually very well controlled in commercial poultry production. Dermatophytosis caused by *Microsporum gallinae* is known as favus but is only seen rarely, and a range of other fungi have also been associated with dermatitis (Pass, 1989). 'Scaly leg' caused by *Cnemidocoptes mutans* is associated with obvious thickening of the scaled epidermis of the lower leg, rarely seen in commercial poultry production but more commonly in small flocks. Ironically it is other mites, *Dermanyssus gallinae* in particular, that are the most challenging to control and have the greatest impact. In addition to causing marked anaemia, they cause substantial flock disturbance and can act as a trigger for injurious pecking; they can even act as vectors of important systemic infectious diseases, especially *Salmonella gallinarum*, but perhaps others also.

Viral and bacterial infections

In commercial poultry the classic diseases affecting skin are those caused by Avipox virus (fowlpox lesions can also extend into the mouth, pharynx and larynx) and the skin form of Marek's disease, which was a common finding in broilers at slaughter prior to the implementation of effective control measures for this condition.

Systemic bacterial infections can result from traumatic damage to skin. Erysipelas is commonly associated with infection of scratches or wounds (in humans and sheep) and the author has observed increased severity of this infection in commercial layers with poor feather coverage and skin damage. Staphylococcal tenosynovitis in broiler parents in rear is commonly seen during the period of maximum feed restriction. Careful management during this period to minimize toe-scratching is helpful in controlling this condition. It has been shown recently that systemic staphylococcal infections can also originate via invasion of contact dermatitis lesions on the feet of broiler parents (Thøfner *et al.*, 2016).

Necrotic dermatitis is attributed to *Clostridium septicum* and/or *Staphylococcus* spp. invasion of the skin and subcutaneous tissues of both meat chickens and turkeys. This may be initiated by traumatic interruption of the integrity of the skin but is also believed to be affected by immunosuppression. In broilers this condition has been seen particularly in birds with low maternal antibody exposed to infectious bursal disease virus in early life. A form of this condition is also seen in progeny of chicken flocks sero-converting to chicken anaemia virus during the laying period (so called blue-wing disease).

Pseudomonas-associated dermatitis/cellulitis has also been described by various authors (Pass, 1989). The mechanism of infection is not always obvious but can include wound infection, inoculation (contaminated vaccine) and probably the conjunctival route (when water is heavily contaminated and supplied in bell drinkers). Young chicks accidentally inoculated with *Pseudomonas* sp. (in contaminated Marek's vaccine diluent) may die within 24 h from septicaemia without obvious gross lesions at the site of inoculation if the infection dose is high, but develop cellulitis at the site of inoculation if the infection loading is lower, allowing survival for a few days. Localized *Pasteurella multocida*-associated cellulitis is commonly seen in the wattles, particularly when fowl cholera occurs in male broiler parents.

Escherichia coli strains can also be associated with wound infections and particular strains seem to be prone to inducing dermatitis/cellulitis of abdominal tissues of broilers (Ngeleka *et al.*, 1996). This condition is a significant component of carcass rejects and has been referred to as 'inflammatory process' in North America. The entry portals are small scratches which typically occur in weeks 3–4 of life when feather cover of that area is still not well established. Ironically, efforts to control contact dermatitis by encouraging dry litter may increase the risk of this condition, because the claws are then cleaner and sharper.

ISSUES AND DISEASES ASSOCIATED WITH THE BEAK

The beak tends to cause few problems in well nourished birds, other than the damage it occasionally causes other birds. We do not currently recognize anything like circovirus-associated psittacine beak and feather disease in farmed poultry. Developmental defects are occasionally seen, either at day-old or later, resulting in twisted beaks or overgrowth of the lower mandible (shovel beak). Affected birds show a surprising ability to adapt to the disability associated with this.

There has been progressively less reliance on surgical interventions to curtail beak growth or achieve blunting for the prevention of cannibalism as a result of a broad range of strategies. A recent review in the UK advised the government that day-old infrared beak treatment should continue to be allowed for the present. This technique is currently carried out on a significant proportion of laying chickens and has been shown to reduce the risk of cannibalism and reduce mortality during the productive life of the birds. Because the treated area of beak is retained for 10–14 days the procedure has minimal impact on chick liveability. In the early years of implementing this technology there were some issues with accumulation of feed dust impacted into the treated area of the upper beak associated with poorer adaptation ('starting') and increased risk of bacterial infections. This issue is avoided by ensuring good access to drinking water and avoiding excessive 'fines' in the starter diet.

ISSUES AND DISEASES ASSOCIATED WITH THE FEATHERS

Feather loss is a natural phenomenon, but can also be a significant health and welfare issue for poultry flocks. Poorly feathered birds in cold climates require more energy in order to maintain body temperature and so feed efficiency is reduced. As discussed elsewhere in this volume, causes of feather loss are diverse and not easily attributed to one specific cause. In many circumstances, careful attention to bird behaviour and good management at all stages of production can help to minimize issues.

The classic feather condition in chickens is 'clubbed-down syndrome' in which feather development in day-old chicks is delayed and many of the feathers remain enclosed in their sheath. Riboflavin deficiency is known to cause this, but even 30 years ago (Pass, 1989) it was already clear that this was not always the cause. This condition is associated with very poor liveability of the progeny of a particular breeding flock and this may continue for a few weeks or for an extended period. It can occur in both meat and egg type chickens. It has been postulated that infection of the parents with particular astroviruses may be involved and this may alter mineral metabolism. Use of chelated trace minerals in the parents is reported to be helpful. There is a much clearer association of another feather syndrome of day-old meat chickens with astrovirus infection (Smyth, 2017). In this case successive hatches over a number of weeks have loss of the normal yellow down colour – so-called 'white chick syndrome'.

Other acute viral infections in young chicks have been associated with disturbances of feather growth, no doubt in part because of the effects of these conditions on nutrient absorption and metabolism. Early viral enteritis resulting in runting–stunting syndrome causes weaknesses and breakages of torsions of feather shafts, particularly of primary and secondary wing feathers, giving the affected chicks a 'helicopter' appearance. Infection with reticuloendotheliosis virus has been associated with a severe feather defect in which barbs are adherent to the rachis, referred to as 'nakanuke'.

We regularly see relatively minor feather defects, particularly close to the feather tips on wing feathers of young chicks, but sometimes also in older birds, of various strains of both meat and egg-producing chickens. These are, typically, transverse bars with a line of used or poorly formed barbules extending at right angles to the vane. It has long been recognized that in wild birds there is a degree of barring due to feather formed at night being slightly different to that in the daytime. It has been proposed to use this effect as the basis of 'ptilochronology' to study nutritional status in a manner analogous to dendrochronology using tree rings (Grubb, 2006). Whether a more detailed study of feather barring in commercial poultry could provide a better understanding of health and welfare during periods of rapid feather growth remains to be seen.

SKIN ISSUES IN SLAUGHTER POULTRY

A significant proportion of poultry meat is sold either as whole carcasses or skin-on portions, and so diseases of, or even cosmetic changes to, the skin can be economically important. The majority of skin blemishes relate to processing issues such as method of slaughter, bleeding efficiency, excessive scalding, physical contamination, tears and bruising (for examples, see Anonymous, 2014; Tondeur *et al.*, 2011). Handling on loading and unloading, and environmental conditions in transport can also have an impact on skin appearance, in particular in relation to congestion and bruising.

CONCLUSIONS

The skin can be affected by inflammation associated with viruses with a tropism for skin (such as poxviruses), and generalized viruses such as Marek's disease, mould infections, and external parasites as well as specific bacterial infections. Physical damage to the integument, whatever the cause, can lead to localized infections in skin, dermis and sub-cutis as well as systemic infection. The consequences of skin damage will vary according to the type and physiological status of the birds, the severity and location of damage and the immune competence of the host.

The integumentary system of poultry can provide useful information to help to improve management and monitor and control specific diseases, thereby maintaining and improving health, welfare and productivity of farmed poultry.

REFERENCES

Anonymous (2014) *Broiler Carcass Condemnation and Downgrade Management Pocket Guide.* Available at: http://eu.aviagen.com/assets/Tech_Center/BB_Resources_Tools/Pocket_Guides/AA-Carcass-Condemned-Pocket-Guide-0714-EN.pdf (accessed 8 October 2018).

Grubb, T.C. (2006) *Ptilochronology: Feather Time and the Biology of Birds.* Oxford Ornithology Series. Oxford University Press, Oxford, UK.

Ngeleka, M., Kwaga, J.K., White, D.G., Whittam, T.S., Riddell, C. *et al.* (1996) *Escherichia coli* cellulitis in broiler chickens: clonal relationships among strains and analysis of virulence-associated factors of isolates from diseased birds. *Infection and Immunity* 64(8), 3118–3126.

Pass, D.A. (1989) The pathology of the avian integument: a review. *Avian Pathology* 18, 1–72. doi: 10.1080/03079458908418580.

Smyth, V.J. (2017) A review of the strain diversity and pathogenesis of chicken astrovirus. *Viruses* 9(2), 29.

Thøfner, I., Poulsen, L.L., Olsen, R.H., Christensen, H., Bisgaard, M. and Christensen, J.P. (2016) Infections with Gram positive cocci in broiler breeders: significance and prevalence. In: *16th International Conference on Production Diseases in Farm Animals: Book of Abstracts.* Wageningen Academic Publishers, Wageningen, Netherlands, s. 141–141. doi: 10.3920/978-90-8686-831-5.

Tondeur, W., Lopéz-Brea, F. and Serrano Masip, X. (2011) Carcass abnormalities in broilers: an Iberian case. In: *Proceedings of the XLVIII Scientific Symposium on Poultry Production – WPSA Spain (AECA).* Available at: http://www.wpsa-aeca.com/aeca_imgs_docs/Tondeur%20Carcass%20abnormalities%20Iberia%202011.pdf

PART III

Genetics

CHAPTER 8
Genetics of Feather Pigmentation and Chicken Plumage Colouration

Victor E. Olori*

Aviagen Ltd, Newbridge, Scotland

ABSTRACT

The chicken's plumage is defined by the structure and colour of its feathers. Plumage colour is a feature used in modern poultry breeding to distinguish between breeds, strains and pure lines. It is therefore important in strain security. Sex-linked genes affecting plumage colour and patterns and rate of feather development are useful in sexing of day-old chicks. Variation in plumage colour is attributable to differences in the primary and secondary colour patterns exhibited by individual birds. While the primary pattern refers to the distribution of coloured feathers in different parts of the bird's body, the secondary pattern refers to the distribution of colour on individual feathers. Although many commercial broiler and layer chicken strains exhibit solid or single colours, the chicken, like many other birds, exhibits a very wide array of plumage colour patterns, due to the presence or absence of pigments on the feathers. While some birds exhibit complete lack of pigment either in individual feathers or in all of the feathers across the body and are hence completely white, others are pigmented and exhibit a range of colours such as black, blue, brown and orange. While some have all their feathers of the same colour (solid colouration), others show a mixture of colours, which may be distributed in a specific pattern in different parts of the body such as the neck, wing and tail feathers, or have multicoloured feathers. It is now clear that all of these colour patterns are under genetic control. The development of pure lines and commercial crosses with specific colour patterns therefore requires a good understanding of the genetics of feather pigmentation and hence the inheritance of plumage colouration. This review highlights current knowledge of the genes that affect colour development and distribution in chickens as well as the pigments that colour feathers and the mechanism of their secretion. It aims to enrich our understanding of the link

*veolori@aviagen.com

between the genes and the causal mutations that affect colour in chickens and the physiological pathways involved in pigment production and distribution between and within feathers of the chicken plumage.

INTRODUCTION

Feathers are a major feature of the integument of birds. They are a specialized derivative of the integument (Stettenheim, 2000) which helps to protect the skin from the physical environment as well as vagaries of the weather. They are useful for thermoregulation as well as for flight, depending on species. The plumage is defined by the structure and colour of the feathers; and variation in feather colour and patterns makes birds one of the most colourful animal species on earth. This is true for domesticated birds like chickens, turkeys and ducks used in poultry production, as it is for wild birds. Even though most crosses of chickens seen in commercial poultry production have solid white, brown or black plumage colours, there is a much bigger variation in colour patterns in pure lines as well as traditional breeds and crosses kept by most breeders and fanciers. Generally, traditional breeds of poultry exhibit an array of plumage colours that match the variation observed across birds. The extent of this variability is most obvious today amongst indigenous chickens used in free-range or semi-extensive poultry production systems where uncontrolled breeding, absence of selection and random mating have facilitated the maintenance of heterogeneity in the numerous loci (Somes, 1980) responsible for plumage feather colouration in chickens.

The evolution of plumage colour patterns, from the relatively simple patterns of the ancestral breeds, has no doubt gone hand in hand with the evolution of domestic chicken from the multiple ancestral species, i.e. the red junglefowl (*Gallus gallus*) from South-East Asia, the Ceylon junglefowl (*Gallus lafeyetti*) from Sri Lanka, the green junglefowl (*Gallus varius*) from Indonesia and the grey junglefowl (*Gallus soneratti*) of India (Crawford, 1990; Liu *et al.*, 2006). Because plumage colour is controlled by numerous genes segregating in the population, its evolution is subject to natural evolutionary forces of dispersion with human migration, isolation, mutation and random breeding. It is also subject to human evolutionary impact such as crossbreeding, selection and inbreeding by the fanciers, exhibitionists and commercial breeders leading to the array of plumage colours and feather patterns in the modern chickens of today. This being the case, one can assume that the ancestral species were segregating for most of the numerous gene loci (Somes, 1980) that contribute to feather colour development and distribution.

Early developers of traditional breeds of chicken used plumage colours extensively as a distinguishing feature of their breeds, especially in the presentation of 'show grade' or award-winning examples of the breed (Jeffrey, 1977). In this regard, plumage colour continues to play a major role for people breeding fancy chickens as a hobby as well as those tasked with maintenance and conservation of these traditional breeds for future generations. It is easily a good indicator of how much selection has taken place within a population of chickens, hence a useful tool in the conservation of chicken genetic resource.

The development of modern solid-coloured strains of chicken for commercial production has been made possible mostly because there is no significant negative pleiotropic or epistatic effect of colour genes on fitness or performance traits of economic interest. In his review of the subject, Mundy (2005) concluded that the melanocortin-1 receptor (MC1-R), the main locus associated with feather colour pigment synthesis in chickens (Takeuchi *et al.*, 1996; Ling *et al.*, 2003), could be used to change plumage colouration without any deleterious impact on other features that constitute the phenotype of the bird. This fact has been exploited by modern poultry breeders in developing commercial crosses of chicken with colours based mostly on aesthetics, customer preference, strain identity and security.

As simple as this may seem, selection for plumage colour and development of a strain or breed that breeds true for a given colour pattern, either for commercial poultry production, exhibition or as a hobby, requires a deep understanding of the extent of plumage colour variation in the population, what causes the observed variability and the mode of inheritance. Such understanding must start with knowledge of what impacts colour on feathers and what affects the distribution or restriction of colour to different feathers or parts of body, such as within individual feathers. An understanding of how the genetic component of plumage colouration in chickens is inherited is pertinent and is the object of this review.

IMPORTANCE OF PLUMAGE COLOUR

The primary role of the integument is to protect the bird from the vagaries of the environment and weather and feathers play a key role in this. The addition of colour pigment strengthens keratins, which are the building blocks of the feather. Melanin, which is the main feather colour pigment, makes feathers resistant to abrasion, allowing them to perform the key role of protecting the birds. In many bird species, visual signals from the plumage and other structures of the epidermis are important for sexual and other social behaviours (Stettenheim, 2000). Plumage colour is therefore important for communication between birds, reproductive success, safety from predators and safety from physical injury. It also helps in protection from parasites and other predatory animals via concealment or show of aggression.

Plumage colour is perhaps the most important feature of the birds amongst traditional breeders, as it confers an aesthetic value on the birds that is desired by fanciers and hobbyists. In the breeding of show birds, plumage colour is a key trait of economic importance and key standard for accurate breed and variety description (Jeffrey, 1977). In modern poultry breeding for commercial production, plumage colour is useful in breed identification and plays an important role in the security of commercial crosses.

Auto-sexing

The most important use of feather colour in commercial chicken breeding is in sexing of day-old chicks. Prominent genes in this regard are the sex-linked 'Barring' gene (B/b^{+}) and the sex-linked 'Silver/gold' gene (S/s^{+}). The barring allele (B) is dominant over the non-barring allele (b), hence individuals with a single B allele are barred. Females are the hemizygous sex in birds with the Z/w sex chromosome pair. Only the Z sex chromosome can harbour a gene, while the second chromosome in the pair, w, does not (Smith *et al.*, 2009). A barred female will therefore have a single ($B/–$) allele while a non-barred female will be ($b/–$). Since a female can only pass her single Z chromosome to her male offspring, she will surely pass the only barring allele she carries to her male offspring. A non-barred male will have only the recessive alleles in a homozygous state ($b+/b+$), hence when a non-barred male is crossed with a barred female, all the male offspring will be barred ($B/b+$) with a black dot on the head at day-old. All the resulting female offspring will be non-barred ($b/–$) and hence will not have a black dot on their head. Table 8.1 illustrates the possible genotypes of male and female offspring resulting from a cross between a barred female and a non-barred male. The presence or absence of the black dot on the head at day-old is used to distinguish males from female chicks at day-old using the barring gene (Nicholson, 2012).

In the same way, Table 8.2 shows the use of the sex-linked Silver/gold gene in auto-sexing. In this case the silver allele (S) is dominant over the wild-type gold allele (s^{+}). Therefore a solid gold male will have the gold allele in a homozygous state (s^{+}/s^{+}) while a silver (or white) female will carry the (S) gene in a hemizygous state ($S/–$). When these are crossed the male offspring will be

Table 8.1. The use of the Barring gene[a] in sex determination in chickens.

Sire: Solid Black or Red (b/b)		Dam: Barred (B/–)	
		Z (*B*)	*W* (–)
		Male (Barred)	Female (Solid)
	$Z(b^{+})$	Z^{B}/Z^{b+}	Z^{b+}/W^{-}
		Male (Barred)	Female (Solid)
	$Z(b^{+})$	Z^{B}/Z^{b+}	Z^{b+}/W^{-}

[a]*B/b+* males are barred with a black dot on head at day-old; *b+/–* females are solid coloured.

Table 8.2. The use of the Silver/Gold[a] locus in sex determination in chickens.

Sire: Solid Gold (s^{+}/s^{+})		Dam: Silver (S/–)	
		Z (*S*)	*W* (–)
		Male (Silver)	Female (Gold)
	$Z(s^{+})$	$Z^{S}/Zs+$	Z^{s+}/W^{-}
		Male (Silver)	Female (Gold)
	$Z(s^{+})$	Z^{S}/Z^{s+}	Z^{s+}/W^{-}

[a]*S/s+* males are silver with light coloured down at day-old while *s+/–* females are gold with dark brown down feathers at day-old.

heterozygous (S/s^+) and with light down-feather colour at day-old while the females will be ($s^+/-$) with dark brown down feather at day-old, thus facilitating the separation of males from females at day-old. These are the mechanism and genes commonly used in the layer breeding industry to sex chicks at day-old (Nicholson, 2012).

Although not related to feather colouring, a similar sex-linked gene, commonly used for sexing day-old chicks in broiler breeding, is the slow-feathering gene K, which is dominant over the recessive wild-type k^+ responsible for fast feathering. A fast-feathering male is homozygous for the recessive form while a slow-feathering female will have the $K/-$ genotype. When these are crossed, all resulting male offspring will be slow feathering (K/k^+) with short primary wing feathers, while all resulting females will be fast feathering ($k^+/-$) with much longer primary wing feathers (Nicholson, 2012).

PLUMAGE COLOUR VARIATION IN THE POPULATION

The chicken's plumage is defined by the structure and colour of its feathers. Plumage colour therefore refers to the colouration and distribution of coloured feathers over the body of the bird. Variation in plumage colour is attributable to differences in the primary and secondary colour patterns exhibited by individual birds. While the primary pattern refers to the distribution of coloured feathers in different parts of the bird's body, the secondary pattern refers to the distribution of colour on individual feathers. The first cause of variation is, therefore, the colour on the feathers and this depends primarily on the presence or absence of colour pigment and the type of pigment present. Plumage colour can also be due to the structure of the feather barbules, which interacts with light and air to produce iridescent and non-iridescent colour hues generally referred to as structural colour (Prum *et al.*, 1994, 1998; Galván and Solano, 2016).

Colour patterns

Plumage colour patterns are created by the distribution of, or restriction of, colour pigments to feathers in different parts of the bird. Figure 8.1 shows a typical male chicken and the types of feathers found in different parts of the body which can be differentially coloured. A bird is said to have solid colouration when all the feathers in the different parts of the body have the same single colour. Solid colours are common patterns in modern commercial chicken breeding where birds are either all white (such as many broilers breeds), brown (most layer breeds) or black. A bird is said to exhibit 'primary colour pattern' when all the feathers in certain parts of the body are of the same colour and different from the colour of the feathers in a different part of the body. If, on the other hand, colour pigments are restricted to certain parts of the individual feathers such as the tip or edge only, or different colour pigments are deposited in different parts of the feathers, then the bird is said to exhibit the secondary plumage pattern. Thus even when a bird has the pigment to impart a single colour, the distribution

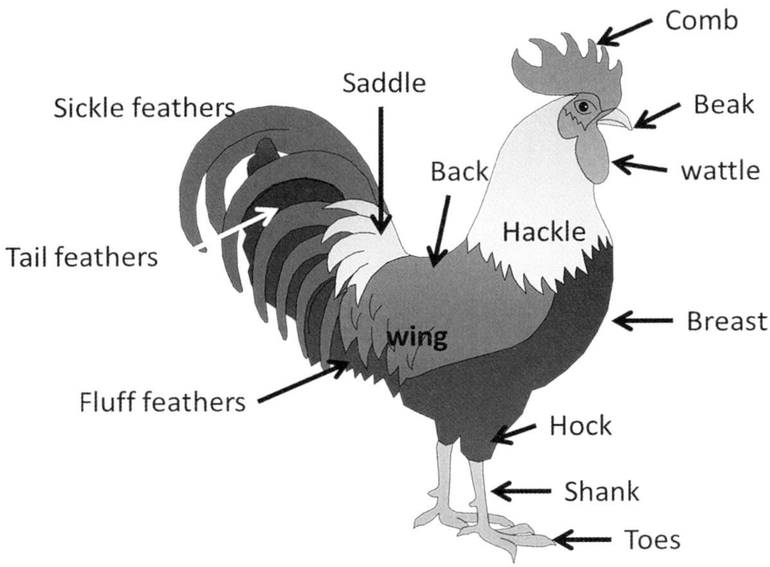

Fig. 8.1. Feathers of the different parts of the chicken.

or restriction of the pigments to different feathers or parts of the feather alone can lead to variation in the plumage colour.

Figure 8.2 shows a bird with solid black colour (a) compared with one with a primary pattern due to restriction of black colour to certain parts of the body (b) and another where black colour is restricted to certain parts of all the feathers of the body (c).

FEATHER COLOUR PIGMENTS AND THEIR SYNTHESIS

The primary colour pigments found in chicken feathers are the melanins (Takeuchi *et al.*, 1996; Ling *et al.*, 2003; McGraw *et al.*, 2004; Mundy, 2005; Roulin and Ducrest, 2013; Galván and Solano, 2016). Other pigments found,

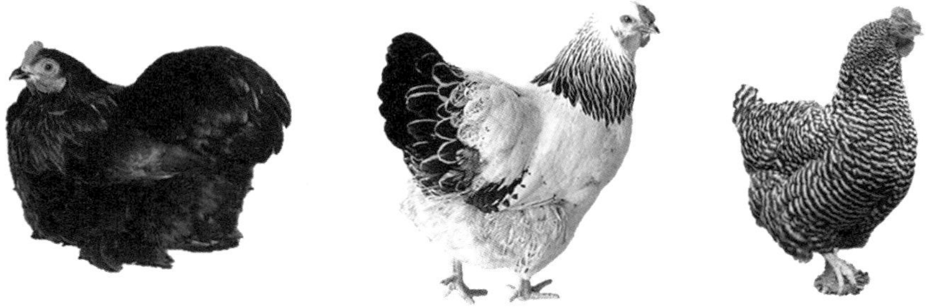

Fig. 8.2. Birds with a solid (a) primary pattern (b) and secondary pattern; (c) plumage colour based on only the black colour.

mostly in other bird species and in other integumentary tissues, include carotenes, porphyrins, flavins and psittacofulvin (polyene lipochrome), pterins, purines and turacin (Brush, 1990; McGraw *et al.*, 2004; McGraw and Klasing, 2006; Roulin and Ducrest, 2013; Galván and Solano, 2016). Melanins are heterogeneous natural polymers produced by the melanosome organelles in melanocyte cells. In birds, the melanosomes are transferred to the cytoplasm of keratinocyte cells as the feather forms and grow from the dermal papillae with keratin deposition (Galván and Solano, 2016).

There are two main types of melanin found in birds. These are eumelanin, which imparts black and grey colouration, and phaeomelanin, which is responsible for reddish and brown colouration (Takeuchi, *et al.*, 1996; Ling *et al.*, 2003; McGraw *et al.*, 2004; Mundy, 2005; Roulin and Ducrest, 2013; Galván and Solano, 2016). Other colours and hues can be attributed to pigment enhancement, dilution, or mixture as well as structural colour. The two types of melanin pigments are produced in structurally different, dedicated organelles or melanosomes during melanogenesis (Galván and Solano, 2016). This process is catalysed by tyrosinase (Tyr), which is a rate-limiting enzyme. Although these pigments are derived from a common precursor (L-tyrosine and L-dopaquinone), their synthesis follows different pathways and may depend on how much tyrosinase enzyme, tyrosinase-related proteins (Trp1) and other precursors such as L-cysteine and cysteinyl-dopa is present (Roulin and Ducrest, 2013; Galván and Solano, 2016).

Melanogenesis, and how much of eumelanin or phaeomelanin pigments are produced, is under the control of the melanocortin-1 receptor (MC1-R) (Takeuchi *et al.*, 1996; Ling *et al.*, 2003; Mundy, 2005; Roulin and Ducrest, 2013). This receptor is a member of the transmembrane G protein-coupled receptors that is expressed in melanocytes and believed to be well conserved across many vertebrate species (Kijas *et al.*, 1998; Schiöth *et al.*, 2005). Melanin production is triggered when melanin-stimulating hormone (α-MSH) binds to the MC1-R, leading to the production of cyclic adenosine monophosphate (cAMP). This is a second messenger that induces the production of the microphthalmia-associated transcription factor (MITF) (Shibahara *et al.*, 2001) and increases activity of Tyr, Tryp1 and other proteins involved in melanogenesis. How much and which melanin pigment is produced depends on the level of tyrosinase activity. High levels of tyrosinase activity lead to increased production of eumelanin, while low levels of tyrosinase activity result in production of phaeomelanin (Liu *et al.*, 2010; Xu *et al.*, 2013). Therefore, factors that control the synthesis, availability and function of the precursors, hormones, enzymes, metal ions and proteins involved in the melanin synthesis pathway are implicated in the control of melanogenesis. These thus affect the synthesis and quantity of eumelanin relative to phaeomelanin produced, which eventually determine the colour of the bird.

GENETIC CONTROL OF PIGMENT SYNTHESIS

The control of melanin synthesis is dependent on genetic and non-genetic factors. For example, diet and available dietary amino acids could influence plumage colour (Poston *et al.*, 2005) because they affect the availability of proteins such as cysteine, phenylalanine and tyrosine precursor, all of which are important in melanin synthesis. Environmental constraints limiting the availability of all or some of these basic requirements of melanogenesis have been shown to impact plumage colour in a wild bird species (Galván *et al.*, 2010). Genetic factors exert by far the most diverse control on bird colouration via their influence on melanogenesis in birds. This influence is mediated via genes that code for highly specific enzymes such as tyrosinase, structural and regulatory proteins such as the intra-melanosomal protein (PMel) (Mochii *et al.*, 1991; Martínez-Esparza *et al.*, 1999), membrane transporters such as cAMP and MITF, hormones such as α-MSH as well as receptors such as MC1-R, all of which are involved in melanin biosynthesis (Galván and Solano, 2016). Eumelanin is structurally different from phaeomelanin and these pigments are produced from structurally different melanocytes (Galván and Solano, 2016; Kijas *et al.*, 1998). In general, about 120 genes have been implicated in the genetic control of coat colour in animals (Chintala *et al.*, 2005), of which about 50 have been associated with colour determination in birds (Somes, 1980; Van Grouw, 2013).

MODE OF ACTION OF GENES AFFECTING FEATHER COLOUR

The variation of plumage colour seen in the population is due primarily to the presence or absence of pigment, enhancement or dilution of pigment and restriction of pigment. These also underline the effect of the different genes that have been associated with feather colouration in birds. The most comprehensive list of these was presented by Somes (1980). The modes of action or effects of these different genes also serve as means to classify the genes in order to understand the complex effect on plumage colour. Van Grouw (2013) described a method of classifying the gene mutations into groups based on their effect and defined the most common effects as 'albinism', 'leucism', 'brown', 'dilution', 'ino' and 'melanism'. While albinism is attributable to a single autosomal recessive gene (*c*) and brown which is also known as 'gold' is due to a single sex-linked recessive gene, the other modes of action are each controlled by a group of genes (Van Grouw and de Jong, 2009).

While 'albinism' refers to complete absence of melanin from feathers, skin and eyes, 'leucism' refers to the partial or complete absence of melanin from feathers and skin only. It thus includes variations due to the effect of patterning genes. The 'brown' gene effect is attributable to a qualitative reduction of eumelanin due to incomplete formation when the eumelanin is not fully oxidized. This form results in plumage colour that is susceptible to bleaching by the sun as the bird ages (Van Grouw, 2013). When both eumelanin and phaeomelanin are synthesized incompletely, i.e. both are not completely oxidized, there is the 'ino' form of gene action. So while both 'brown' and 'ino' forms of gene action involves qualitative reduction in melanin due to incomplete oxidation, the 'brown' form involves only eumelanin while the 'ino' form involves both melanins.

The 'dilution' gene action is due to a quantitative reduction in both melanin pigments resulting in a pale or weaker colouration. The final form ('melanism') refers to a group of genes that cause abnormal deposition of melanin, resulting in increased intensity of black or reddish-brown colouration. This includes the group of colour-enhancing genes. Although Van Grouw (2013) described these modes of action in general using wild bird species, they have similar application in describing the mode of action of colour genes in chickens.

THE COLOUR GENERATION 'EXTENDED BLACK' LOCUS

Several studies have shown that, like the 'Extension' locus in mammals, the 'Extended black' locus in birds (*E*/*e*+) is by far the most significant single locus affecting feather colour in birds (Smyth, 1994; Takeuchi *et al.*, 1996; Ling *et al.*, 2003). It is described as the 'primary feather pattern' locus in the alphabetical list of genes of the domestic fowl compiled by Somes (1980). Mundy (2005) showed via a candidate gene approach that the MC1-R locus alone was responsible for melanin polymorphism. Earlier, Ling *et al.* (2003) had made the link between different MC1-R and different alleles of the *E* locus, confirming the findings of studies that demonstrated distinct structural differences between the MC1 receptors associated with the different alleles of the *E* locus (Takeuchi *et al.*, 1996; Guo *et al.*, 2010). These two studies showed conclusively the link between the different alleles of the *E* locus and how they control the biosynthesis of melanin. We now know that the type of melanocytes present, which determine the type of melanin produced, vary with type of MC1-R receptor. The structure and function of the MC1-R depends on the allele of the *E* locus in the genotype of the bird. So, while level of tyrosinase activity determines how much of eumelanin versus phaeomelanin is produced, its activity is dependent on suitable binding sites, which are controlled by the type of MC1-R present. This receptor is determined by the allele of the extended black (E/e^+) locus.

Extensive work done by many early pioneers in feather colour genes which helped identify the alleles of the 'Extended black' locus was reviewed by Smyth (1965). The most common alleles that have been described for the 'Extended black' locus (Somes, 1980; Smyth, 1994; Ling *et al.*, 2003) are presented in Table 8.3. The order of dominance is E, E^R, $E^{Rfayoumi}$, e^{wh}, e^+, e^b and e^y, indicating that the alleles that produced eumelanin (hence black and grey colouration) are dominant over those that produce phaeomelanin (brownish and red colouration). The final phenotypic expression of plumage colour and pattern, however, will depend on the sex of the bird (Ling *et al.*, 2003) as well as the genotype with regards to the *E* locus and other colour loci which affect the expression of alleles present at the *E* locus.

Amino acid sequence of MC1-R derived from different alleles of the *E* locus indicate that the difference between the wild type allele (*e*+) and the others is a single mutation of Glutamine (Glu) in the wild type (*e*+) to Lysine (Lys) in position 92 of the chromosome. Other differences in amino acid composition have been reported by Ling *et al.* (2003).

Table 8.3. Common alleles of the 'Extended black' locus (E/e^+).

Locus/Allele	Description/Action
E (Extended Black)	Autosomal dominant; allows production of eumelanin for black pigmentation. E/E genotype results in solid black colour depending on the effect of other loci with epistatic effect on E/E
E^R (Birchen) $E^{RFayoumi}$	Produces black colouration but allows phaeomelanin extension to some areas. Hence typically male birds have silver or gold areas in hackles, saddles and shoulders, but only around the neck for females. The $E^{RFayoumi}$ is a special case of this found in Fayoumi breed of chickens
e^+ (Duckwing)	This allele is the wild type of the extended black locus with many varieties, including e^{Wh}, e^b and e^y. It is recessive and sexually dimorphic in expression. Males with all varieties look similar, with black breast and red feathers on hackle and saddle. Females have stippled brown feathers on the back and wings and salmon-coloured feathers on the breast
e^{Wh} (Wheaten) e^y	Extends phaeomelanin and restricts eumelanin in some areas. Adults males are black breasted and red in the rest of the body; adult females are wheaten or have lighter shades of brown with any black colour restricted to the wing and tail feathers, depending on other loci
e^b (Brown or Partridge)	Extends dark brown areas over black areas allowed by $e+$

ABSENCE OF COLOUR (SOLID WHITE PLUMAGE GENOTYPES)

While the E locus determines which pigment is produced, other loci affect how much of the pigment is produced, thereby enhancing the colour. Yet others restrict pigment production to some feathers or parts of the feather, resulting in primary and secondary colour patterns, or dilute the colour of the pigment partially or completely. When the synthesized black or brown pigment is completely diluted or its production is completely restricted, the result is a bird in which all feathers are white with a solid white plumage. There are two major loci responsible for solid white plumage colours in chickens. These are the recessive white ($C+/c$) and the dominant white loci (I^+/i).

Recessive white (C^+, c, c^a, c^{re})

The most notorious locus restricting pigment production is the autosomal recessive gene A^+/a, also referred to as autosomal albinism. The homozygous recessive form (a/a) prevents the production of any pigment, leading to a completely (solid) white plumage colour. Silversides and Crawford (1990) described another mutation ($S^{al\text{-}s}$) which causes imperfect albinism in chickens. However, birds with the more common autosomal albinism genotype have no colour pigment in the eye and other integuments. The resulting pink eye of the birds with autosomal albinism is what distinguishes them from birds with solid white plumage due to other gene loci. It is now widely accepted that autosomal albinism is one of three mutant alleles at the recessive white locus (C^+/c) generally referred to as the 'Tyrosinase gene' (Tobita-Teramoto *et al.*, 2000). The other alleles are c^{re} for red-eye white, c^a for the autosomal albinism and *c* for the recessive white. When the recessive allele is present in the homozygous form (*c/c*), both eumelanin and phaeomelanin pigments are changed to white in the feathers but not in the eye. The dominant wild type C^+, on the other hand, allows colour production depending on which melanin pigment is produced.

A sequence of the tyrosinase cDNA of white chickens with the autosomal recessive gene (c^a/c^a) has shown that the lack of pigment production is associated with tyrosinase inactivity due to two silent point mutations and a six base-pair deletion at position 817 of the tyrosinase gene (Tobita-Teramoto *et al.*, 2000). Mapping of the tyrosinase gene of the recessive white *c/c* indicated that the recessive white phenotype in chickens was due to an avian retroviral sequence insertion in intron 4 of the tyrosinase gene (Chang *et al.*, 2006; Sato *et al.*, 2007).

Dominant white (I, i^+, I^D, I^S)

The dominant white is a multi-allelic gene locus which also has the 'Dun' (I^D) and 'Smoky' (I^S) alleles. It is an autosomal gene that confers solid white colouration in the presence of single dominant *I* allele. *I* and I^D alleles inhibit the expression of black colour by inhibiting melanin pigment production in the feathers only. The presence of the Smoky I^S allele partially restores colour, giving the plumage a smoky look with little melanin production. DNA sequence analysis associates the dominant white allele with a 9 bp insertion in exon 10 which causes the insertion of three amino acids in the transmembrane region of the PMel17 protein. The Dun allele (I^D) is associated with a deletion of five amino acids in the transmembrane region, while the Smoky allele (I^S), which shares the 9 bp insertion with the *I* allele in exon 10, also has a 12 bp deletion in exon 6, leading to the loss of four amino acids from the PMel17 protein (Kerje *et al.*, 2004).

COLOUR ENHANCEMENT OR DILUTION GENES

Colour enhancers

These are the genes that help to emphasize or deepen (enhance) or lighten (dilute) colour pigments, resulting in variation in colour shades. The most notable black colour enhancer is the 'Melanotic' gene (Ml/ml^+) (Moore and Smyth, 1971). It is an autosomal incompletely dominant gene, which implies that the heterozygous form (Ml/ml^+) has less penetrance than the homozygous *Ml/Ml*. This gene extends solid black colour to white and brown areas in the presence of the wild-type allele (e^+) which normally does not favour development of black colour. It thus restricts phaeomelanin and extends black eumelanin into more parts of the body. Conversely, a common brown colour-enhancing gene is the 'Mahogany' gene (*Mh*/*mh*$^+$), which partially restricts eumelanin (Black pigment) and enhances or extends phaeomelanin, hence brown/red colouration, into more areas of the body. It is an autosomal dominant gene that intensifies red colour, especially when present in homozygous form. Both *Ml* and *Mh* genes are therefore important in feather colour patterning in chickens.

Colour diluters

Genes that dilute primary colours are essentially genes that are capable of diluting the pigments, making them lose their colour completely or partially, resulting in lighter shades of black (eumelanin diluters) or brown (phaeomelanin diluters). Van Grouw (2013) described three forms of dilution found in birds. The first, termed 'pastel', includes genes that act on both eumelanin and phaeomelanin, leading to almost 50% reduction in intensity, hence resulting in paler shades of the respective black or brown colours. The second form of diluters, referred to as 'isabel', are those that dilute the black pigment (eumelanin) but have no effect on phaeomelanin, the brown pigment. This form is common in brown broilers with splash or white wing feathers. The third form is that typified by the sex-linked dominant Silver gene (*S*/*s*+). It includes genes that have a diluting effect on phaeomelanin but have no effect on eumelanin.

The most aggressive eumelanin diluter is the 'Dominant white' gene (*I*/*i*$^+$), which completely dilutes eumelanin from a black colour to white. Varieties of this allele have varying levels of 'bleaching' effect on eumelanin pigments. I^D dilutes black to a white colour with a brown taint also referred to 'dun', 'fawn' or 'khaki' colouration, perhaps allowing little pheaomelanin production. The I^s variety dilutes black to a smoky colour, the depth of which is dose dependent (Kerje *et al.*, 2004)

The 'Blue feather' locus (*Bl*/*bl*$^+$) is an incompletely dominant autosomal gene which has varying dilution effect on eumelanin. The homozygous *bl*$^+$/*bl*$^+$ genotype has no diluting effect on eumelanin of a typically black genotype bird, hence birds with this genotype will remain black. The heterozygous *Bl*/*bl*$^+$ form dilutes eumelanin to a bluish colour while the homozygous dominant genotype *Bl*/*Bl* dilutes eumelanin almost completely to produce splash or tainted white colouration in feathers that should otherwise be black. The 'Lavender' gene (*Lav*/*lav*$^+$) is an autosomal recessive gene which dilutes both eumelanin and phaeomelanin, resulting in white feather colours with a bluish taint in the homozygous recessive form *lav*$^+$/*lav*$^+$. This dilution results from the presence of pigmented and non-pigmented regions in the feather barb (Mayerson and Brumbaugh, 1981). This gene is associated with a point mutation within the 'Melanophilin' (*MLPH*) gene located on the chicken chromosome 7 which results in amino acid change (R35W) from arginine in the wild type to tryptophan (Vaez *et al.*, 2008). The 'Dilute' gene (*Di*/*di*+) is an incompletely dominant gene that acts primarily as a phaeomelanin diluter, leading to the production of buff or yellowish brown colours.

PLUMAGE PATTERNING GENES

Patterning is the phenomenon in plumage colouration whereby the bird is covered by more than one colour distributed non-randomly across the body of the bird, as against solid colouration whereby the entire plumage is covered by only one colour as seen in Fig. 8.2a. It is due to genes that restrict or extend different colour production to groups of feathers in different parts of the body or different parts of individual feathers. The mode of action of patterning genes does not involve the presence or absence of pigment-producing cells, as melanocytes are evenly distributed in the follicles of both coloured and non-coloured (white) feathers. Instead, colour patterning is believed to result from regulation of melanin synthesis due to non-random activation of MC1-R by extra-cellular ligands involved in melanogenesis in different cells (Gluckman and Mundy, 2017).

Primary plumage pattern

Restriction of different colours to groups of feathers in different parts of the body creates a primary plumage pattern as seen in Fig. 8.2b. This example is due to the 'Columbian' restriction gene (*Co/co+*), which restricts eumelanin production to the hackle and tail feathers, keeping the main areas of the body white or brown (depending on other genotypes). Its mode of action is similar to the 'Dark brown' (Db/db^+) with the exception that while the Columbian gene dilutes red phaeomelanin pigment to a lighter shade in the main parts of the body, the *Db* gene enhances it, giving the bird a deeper shade of brown in the main body. In both cases, eumelanin is restricted to the neck/hackle and tail feathers, making them black while the rest of the body is covered in white or brown feathers. Another example of genes that cause primary patterns in the plumage is the 'Inhibitor of gold' gene (Ig^+/ig). This is an autosomal recessive gene that restricts phaeomelanin but has no impact on melanin. The 'Silver/gold' gene (*S/s+*) is a sex-linked dominant gene that extends white colour to areas with black or gold background. The dominant allele (*S*) dilutes phaeomelanin from gold or red colouration to silver or white, but this gene has no effect on eumelanin (Meijers, 2017).

Secondary patterns

Secondary colour patterns refer to the non-random distribution or restriction of colour to different parts of individual feathers as seen in Fig. 8.2c. This example is caused by the sex-linked dominant 'Barring' gene (B/b^+). It disrupts eumelanin, resulting in horizontal lines of white on individual black or brown feathers. Recent studies (Hellström *et al.*, 2010; Thalmann *et al.*, 2017) have associated sex-linked barring with regulatory mutation in the tumour suppressor gene *CDKN2A*. This involves two mis-sense mutations and two non-coding changes present, depending on the allele. These studies indicate that barring or the white striping is due to premature differentiation, which leads to loss of melanocyte progenitors in the white parts of the feathers. Homozygous *B/B* males have wider white lines compared with heterozygous *B/b+* males and hemizygous *B/–* females with narrower white strips.

Other examples include the 'Lacing' (Lg/lg^{+}) gene which restricts colour to or away from the edge of the feather barb. The 'Pencilling' gene (*Pg/pg+*) results in concentric patterns on feathers, the extent of which depends on the genotype and other genes. Table 8.4 shows examples of secondary pattern genes and their effect. Primary patterns depend on interaction between the pattern genes and other genes that develop, enhance or dilute colour pigments.

Detailed description and pictures of some of these gene effects are well illustrated online by Meijers (2017). Other useful websites that give good illustration of the feather colour genotypes developed for poultry fanciers and breeders are 'FeatherSite' (http://www.feathersite.com/) and the Dutch 'Kippenjungle' (in Dutch or English) (http://kippenjungle.nl/).

Table 8.4. Plumage colour patterning genes in chickens.

Gene/Locus	Name	Description
Primary patterns		
Co/co+	Columbian restriction	Autosomal recessive gene which restricts eumelanin to tail and hackle feathers only while the rest of the body is white
Db/db+	Dark brown	Limits eumelanin and enhances phaeomelanin. So extends brown colouration to white areas. Homozygous *Db/Db* form acts like *Co* by allowing eumelanin and hence black colour in hackle and tail feathers
Ig/ig+	Gold restrictor	
Lav/lav+	Lavender	Autosomal recessive. Adds blue taint on solid white areas. Dilutes phaeomelanin
S/s+	Silver/Gold	Sex-linked dominant. The *S* allele dilutes both eumelanin and phaeomelanin, extending solid white colours to areas that would otherwise have black or brown colour
Mh/mh+	Mahogany	Autosomal dominant. Partial eumelanin restrictor creating primary colour pattern. It enhances phaeomelanin, hence intensifies brown/red colours
Secondary patterns		
Pg/pg+	Pattern Gene or Pencilling gene	Develops different forms of pencilling patterns on individual feathers such as concentric
Lg/lg+	Lacing gene	Restricts colour to or away from the edge of the feather barb
$B\ B^{sd}$, *b+*	Barring	Sex-linked dominant. Disrupts pigments, forming streaks of white horizontal lines on the feather with a black or brown background
Mo/mo+	Mottling gene	Autosomal recessive gene leading to development of random dots of white on a black or brown background
Ma+/ma	Marbling	This gene forms streak of non-horizontal white lines across individual feathers with a black or brown background

SUMMARY

The plumage of the bird is defined by the structure and colour of its feathers. Plumage colour is important for signalling and hence in reproductive success and survival. There are two sources of colour. Structural colour results from the interaction of ordered keratin layers on feather barbules with air and light producing iridescent and non-iridescent colour hues. Most pronounced colouration is due to pigments that are synthesized and added to the feathers as they develop. Pigmentary colour is mostly due to two forms of melanin: (i) eumelanin, which imparts black and grey colouration; and (ii) phaeomelanin, which imparts brown/red colours. Variation in shades and intensity of these colours is due to the action of genes with epistatic effect on the primary pigment locus.

Both forms of melanin are synthesized by specialized melanophores or organelles in the melanocyte cells. Though arising from the same precursors, the synthesis of both pigments follows different pathways, depending on the level of tyrosinase activity. The control of melanogenesis has been associated with melanocortin 1 receptor. Structurally different forms of this receptor have been associated with different alleles of the 'Extended black' *E/e+* locus, which determines which of the melanin pigments is produced.

Further variation in plumage colour is brought about by colour patterning genes that are responsible for the presence of more than one colour in different parts of the body or different parts of each feather. The variation in colour pigment, restriction, extension and dilution of the pigments along with patterning genes are responsible for the wonderful array of colours found in domestic chickens that match what is observed in wild birds.

REFERENCES

Brush, A.H. (1990) Metabolism of carotenoid pigments in birds. *FASEB Journal* 4(12), 2969–2977.

Chang, C.M., Voville, J.L., Coquerelle, G., Gourichon, D., Oulmouden, A. and Tixier-Boichard, M. (2006) Complete association between a retroviral insertion in the tyrosinase gene and the recessive white mutation in chickens. *BMC Genomics* 7, 19. doi: 10.1186/1471-2164-7-19.

Chintala, S., Li, W., Lamoreux, M.L., Ito, S., Wakamatsu, K. *et al.* (2005) Slc7a11 gene controls production of pheomelanin pigment and proliferation of cultured cells. *Proceedings of the National Academy of Sciences USA* 102(31), 10964–10969. doi: 10.1073/pnas.0502856102.

Crawford, R.D. (1990) Origin and history of poultry species. In: Crawford, R.D. (ed.) *Poultry Breeding and Genetics*. Elsevier, Amsterdam, pp. 1–41.

Galván, I. and Solano, F. (2016) Bird integumentary melanins: biosynthesis, forms, function and evolution. *International Journal of Molecular Sciences* 17, 520. doi: 10.3390/ijms17040520.

Galván, I., Bijlsma, R.G., Negro, J.J., Jarén, M. and Garrido-Fernández, J. (2010) Environmental constraints for plumage melanization in the Northern Goshawk (*Accipiter gentilis*). *Journal of Avian Biology* 41, 523–531.

Gluckman, T.L. and Mundy, N.I. (2017) The differential expression of MC1R regulators in dorsal and ventral quail plumages during embryogenesis: implication for plumage pattern formation. *PLOS ONE* 12, e0174714. doi: 10.1371/journal.pone.0174714.

Guo, X.L., Li, X.L., Li, Y., Gu, Z.L., Zheng, C.S. *et al.* (2010) Genetic variation of chicken MC1R gene in different plumage colour populations. *British Poultry Science* 51, 734–739.

Hellström, A.R., Sundström, E., Gunnarsson, U., Bed'Hom, B., Tixier-Boichard, M. *et al.* (2010) Sex-linked barring in chickens is controlled by the CDKN2A/B tumour suppressor locus. *Pigment Cell & Melanoma Research* 2, 3521–3530.

Jeffrey, F.P. (1977) *Bantam Breeding and Genetics.* Spur Publications Company, Hindhead, England.

Kerje, S., Sharma, P., Gunnarsson, U., Kim, H., Bagchi, S. *et al.* (2004) The Dominant white, Dun and Smoky colour variants in chicken are associated with insertion/deletion polymorphisms in the PMEL17 gene. *Genetics* 168(3), 1507–1518. doi: 10.1534/genetics.104.027995

Kijas, J.M.H., Wales, R., Törnsten, A., Chardon, P., Moller, M. and Andersson, L. (1998) Melanocortin receptor 1 (MC1R) mutations and coat color in pigs. *Genetics* 150(3), 1177–1185.

Ling, M.K., Lagerstöm, M.C., Fredriksson, R., Okimoto, R., Mundy, N.I., Takeuchi, S. and Schiölth, H.B. (2003) Association of feather colour with constitutively active melanocortin 1 receptors in chicken. *European Journal of Biochemistry* 270, 1441–1449.

Liu, Y.P., Wu, G.S., Yao, Y.G., Miao, Y.W., Luikart, G. *et al.* (2006) Multiple maternal origins of chickens: out of the Asian jungles. *Molecular Phylogenetics and Evolution* 38, 12–19. doi: 10.1016/j.ympev.2005.09.014

Liu, W.B., Chen, S.R., Zheng, J.X., Qu, L.J., Xu, G.Y. and Yang, N. (2010) Developmental phenotypic-genotypic associations of tyrosinase and melanocortin 1 receptor genes with changing profiles in chicken plumage pigmentation. *Poultry Science* 89, 1110–1114.

Martínez-Esparza, M., Jiménez-Cervantes, C., Bennett, D.C., Lozano, J.A., Solano, F. and García-Borrón, J.C. (1999) The murine silver locus: coding and expression of a single transcript truncated by the silver mutation. *Mammalian Genome* 10, 1168–1171.

Mayerson, P.L. and Brumbaugh, J.A. (1981) Lavender, a chick melanocyte mutant with defective melanosome translocation: a possible role for 10 nm filaments and microfilaments but not microtubules. *Journal of Cell Science* 51, 25–51.

McGraw, K.J. and Klasing, K.C. (2006) Carotenoids, immunity, and intergumentary coloration in Red Jungle fowl (*Gallus gallus*). *The Auk* 123, 1161–1171. doi: 10.1642/0004-8038(2006)123[1161:CIAICI]2.0.CO;2

McGraw, K.J., Wakamatsu, K., Ito, S., Nolan, P.M, Jouventin, P. *et al.* (2004) You can't judge a pigment by its color: carotenoid and melanin content of yellow and brown feathers in swallows, bluebirds, penguins and domestic chickens. *The Condor* 106, 390–395.

Meijers, H.H.M. (2017) *Poultry Mutations: Sub Menu 1.* Available at: http://www.edelras.nl/chickengenetics/mutations1.html (accessed 9 October 2018).

Mochii, M., Agata, K. and Eguchi, G. (1991) Complete sequence and expression of a cDNA encoding a chicken 115-kDa melanosomal matrix protein. *Pigment Cell & Melanoma Research* 4, 41–47.

Moore, J.W. and Smyth, J.R. (1971) Melanotic, key to a phenotypic enigma of the fowl. *Journal of Heredity* 62, 214–219.

Mundy, N.I. (2005) A window on the genetics of evolution: MC1R and plumage colouration in birds. *Proceedings of the Royal Society of London B: Biological Sciences* 272, 1633–1640.

Nicholson, H. (2012) *Genetics Mini-series 6: Sex Linkage.* Available at: https://scratchcradle.wordpress.com/2012/08/05/gms6-sex-linkage/ (accessed 9 October 2018).

Poston, J.P., Hasselquist, D., Stewart, I.R.K. and Westneat, D.F. (2005) Dietary amino acids influence plumage traits and immune responses of male house sparrows, *Passer domesticus*, but not as expected. *Animal Behaviour* 70, 1171–1181.

Prum, R.O., Morrison, R.L. and ten Eyck, G.R. (1994) Structural color production by constructive reflection from ordered collagen arrays in a bird (*Philepitta custanea*: Eurylaimidae). *Journal of Morphology* 222, 61–72.

Prum, R.O., Torres, R.H., Williamson, S. and Dyck, J. (1998) Coherent light scattering by blue bird feather barbs. *Nature* 396, 28–29.

Roulin, A. and Ducrest, A. (2013) Genetics of colouration in birds. *Seminars in Cell & Developmental Biology* 24, 594–608.

Sato, S., Otake, T., Suzuki, C., Saburi, J. and Kobayashi, E. (2007) Mapping of the recessive white locus and analysis of the tyrosinase gene in chickens. *Poultry Science* 86, 2126–2133.

Schiöth, H.B., Haitina, T., Ling, M.K., Ringholm, A., Fredriksson, R., Cerdá-Reverter, J.M. and Klovins, J. (2005) Evolutionary conservation of the structural, pharmacological, and genomic characteristics of the melanocortin receptor subtypes. *Peptides* 26, 1886–1900.

Shibahara, S., Takeda, K., Yasumoto, K., Udono, T., Watanabe, K., Saito, H. and Takahashi, K. (2001) Microphthalmia-associated transcription factor (MITF): multiplicity in structure, function, and regulation. *Journal of Investigative Dermatology Symposium Proceedings* 6, 99–104.

Silversides, F.G. and Crawford, R.D. (1990) Genetic aspects of a new mutation ($S^{al\text{-}s}$) to sex-linked imperfect albinism in chickens. *Genetic Selection Evolution* 22(4), 447–455.

Smith, C.A., Roeszler, K.N., Ohnesorg, T., Cummins, D.M., Farlie, P.G., Doran, T.J and Sinclair, A.H. (2009) The avian Z-linked gene DMRT1 is required for male sex determination in the chicken. *Nature* 461, 267–271.

Smyth, J.R. Jr (1965) Allelic relationship of genes determining extended black, wild type and brown plumage patterns in the fowl. *Poultry Science 44*, 89–98. doi: 10.3382/ps.0440089

Smyth, J.R. (1994) Melanin pigmentation: its biological roles, inheritance and expression in the chicken. *Poultry Science* 73, 106–117.

Somes, R.G. Jr (1980) Alphabetical list of the genes of domestic fowl. *Journal of Heredity* 71, 168–174.

Stettenheim, P.R. (2000) The integumentary morphology of modern birds – an overview. *American Zoologist* 40(4), 461–477. doi: 10.1093/icb/40.4.461

Takeuchi, S., Suzuki, H., Yabuuchi, M. and Takahashi, S. (1996) A possible involvement of melanocortin 1-receptor in regulating feather color pigmentation in the chicken. *Biochimica et Biophysica Acta (BBA) – Gene Structure and Expression* 1308(2), 164–168.

Thalmann, D.S., Ring, H., Sundström, E., Cao, X., Larsson, M. *et al.* (2017) The evolution of Sex-linked barring alleles in chickens involves both regulatory and coding changes in CDKN2A. *PLOS Genetics 13*, e1006665. doi: 10.1371/journal.pgen.1006665.

Tobita-Teramoto, T.J.G.K., Jang, G.Y., Kino, K., Salter, D.W., Brumbaugh, J. and Akiyama, T. (2000) Autosomal albino chicken mutation (ca/ca) deletes hexanucleotide (-?GACTGG817) at a copper-binding site of the tyrosinase gene. *Poultry Science* 79, 46–50.

Vaez, M., Follett, S.A., Bed'hom, B., Gourichon, D., Tixier-Boichard, M. and Burke, T. (2008) A single point-mutation within the melanophilin gene causes the lavender plumage colour dilution phenotype in the chicken. *BioMed Central Genetics* 9, 7. doi: 10.1186/1471-2156-9-7.

Van Grouw, H. (2013) What colour is that bird? The causes and recognition of common colour aberrations in birds. *British Birds* 106, 17–29.

Van Grouw, H. and de Jong, J. (2009) *Genetics in the pigeon, modern Mendelism and more for the pigeon fancier* [in Dutch]. NBS, Surhuisterveen. Cited in: Van Grouw, H. (2017) The dark side of birds: nelanism – facts and fiction. *Bulletin of the British Ornithologist Club* 137, 12–36.

Xu, Y., Zhang, X.H. and Pang, Y.Z. (2013) Association of tyrosinase (TYR) and tyrosinase related protein 1 (TYRP1) with melanic plumage color in Korean quails (*Coturnix coturnix*). *Asian-Australasian Journal of Animal Sciences* 26, 1518–1522.

CHAPTER 9
Genetic and Breeding Aspects of Feather Coverage and Their Effects on Performance in Broilers

Avigdor Cahaner*

The Hebrew University of Jerusalem, Rehovot, Israel

ABSTRACT

Tremendous genetic progress has been achieved in broiler growth rate and meat yield since the 1950s, but it is not fully expressed under hot conditions. Greater growth rate of broilers is driven by greater rates of feed intake and metabolism and elevated production of internal heat. Hot conditions negatively affect high growth-rate broilers by hindering dissipation of the excessive internal heat and elevating body temperature. To avoid heat-induced mortality, broilers acclimate to hot conditions by reducing feed intake, resulting in depressed growth rate and poorer breast meat yield.

The rate of sensible heat dissipation is determined by the insulation of the feathers, which is advantageous in slow-growing chickens or for broilers reared under cool conditions. In high growth-rate broilers under hot conditions, feather coverage hinders the dissipation of excessive internal heat. Hence, it was hypothesized that the negative effects of heat can be alleviated by genes that reduce or eliminate feather coverage. Reduced feather mass was also expected to contribute to greater meat yield, if the saved feather-building proteins were directed to build more muscle mass.

Many studies have been conducted with the co-dominant 'Naked neck' (*Na*) gene that reduces feather coverage by 20% and 40% in *Na*/*na* and *Na*/*Na* chickens, respectively. Under hot conditions, naked-neck broilers exhibit higher rate of heat dissipation, resulting in greater actual growth rate and meat production. However, naked-neck broilers raised at 25°C were superior to their counterparts under hot conditions, indicating that 20–40% reduction in feather coverage provides only partial heat tolerance and suggesting that complete feather elimination is required to maximize heat tolerance.

*avigdor.cahaner@mail.huji.oc.il

To test this hypothesis, the mutation *Scaleless*, which blocks feather formation in *sc/sc* chickens, was introduced into modern high growth-rate broiler stock by backcrossing. The resulting novel experimental line, consisting of featherless broilers and their feathered siblings, had been used in many studies under comfortable versus hot conditions. Under acute heat stress, the featherless birds maintained normal body temperature with no mortality, in contrast to a significant elevation in body temperature of the feathered sibs that led to considerable mortality. In other trials, featherless broilers were compared with feathered sibs under chronic hot conditions (constant 32–35°C) versus comfortable (25°C) conditions. Under heat, only the featherless broilers maintained a normal body temperature, and their mean body weight was significantly higher than their feathered siblings. Under all conditions, the featherless broilers exhibited favourable breast meat yield and quality, apparently due to the saved feather-building nutrients and better vascularization in the breast muscle.

These results indicate that reduction or elimination of feather coverage improved the livability and overall performance of fast-growing broilers in warm and hot conditions.

INTRODUCTION

Remarkable genetic progress has been achieved in broiler growth rate (GR) and meat yield since the 1950s (Havenstein *et al.*, 2003a, b). High GR is driven by high rate of feed intake and metabolism, leading to greater internal heat production (Sandercock *et al.*, 1995). However, the continuously increasing genetic potential for rapid growth and the desirable consequent reduction in time to marketing, with its contribution to better feed efficiency, is not fully expressed under hot conditions (Cahaner, 2008). Hot conditions decrease the difference between ambient temperature (AT) and temperature of the body surface, reducing the rate at which the excessive internal heat is dissipated. The reduced rate of sensible heat loss is stressful at hot conditions because it leads to an elevation in body temperature (BT).

There are two types of heat conditions:

- Acute heat waves: short-term rapid elevation in ambient temperature; elevates body temperature and often leads to mortality. With its sporadic nature and short duration, it is a minor production issue, because mortality can be avoided by feed withdrawal.
- Chronic hot conditions: prevailing year-around in tropical regions and during the hot season in many of broiler-production regions. It is a major global production issue.

Under chronic hot conditions, broilers adapt to heat by reducing feed intake (Cooper and Washburn, 1998; Deeb and Cahaner, 1999, 2001, 2002), but consequently their GR is also reduced, resulting in lower marketing body weight (BW), poorer feed conversion ratio (FCR) and less breast meat (Cahaner and Leenstra, 1992; Leenstra and Cahaner, 1992; Settar *et al.*, 1999).

The response of broilers to hot conditions is defined as one of the two following:

- Heat tolerance: broilers survive the heat, but their productivity is significantly compromised.
- Heat resistance: broilers maintain productivity at normal (maximal) level.

In this text, only heat resistance is considered as a true adaptation to hot conditions.

Hot conditions can be avoided in modern broiler houses that are equipped with efficient cooling systems. However, the global broiler industry continues to expand to hot-climate developing countries where climatic control of broiler houses is limited due to high costs of construction and operation and an unreliable supply of electricity. On the other hand, the need for cooling is increasing, because the stocks of industrial broilers are continuously selected for more rapid growth and higher meat yield and they are reared to higher BW in order to improve the efficiency of mechanical slaughtering and deboning. All these factors are associated with higher metabolism (Sandercock *et al.*, 1995), hence they accentuate the need for enhanced dissipation of the excessive internal heat. Thus, modern broilers need lower AT in order to maintain normal BT and to fully express their genetic potential for rapid growth. With the limited availability of energy and the increasing tendency to minimize the total amount of resources used for human food production, artificial cooling of broiler houses is also becoming an economic and societal burden in developed as well as developing countries. Breeding heat-tolerant broilers may offer a sustainable approach to mitigate the negative effects of heat on broiler production.

In broilers, skin temperature is only 0.5°C lower than BT (Yahav *et al.*, 1997), but due to the thermal resistance (insulation) of the feather coverage, the temperature of the feather-covered body surface is close to AT, hence this surface hardly contributes to the overall sensible heat loss (Cangar *et al.*, 2008). In high-GR broilers under hot conditions, the feather coverage impedes thermoregulation because it hinders sensible heat loss (Yahav *et al.*, 1998; Deeb and Cahaner, 1999). In the 1980s and 1990s, several groups had already tested the hypothesis that the negative effects of high ambient temperatures could be alleviated by introducing genes that reduced or eliminated feather coverage into modern broiler stocks (e.g. Somes and Johnson, 1982; Hanzl and Somes, 1983; Merat, 1986). Other genetic and non-genetic factors may also reduce feather coverage, but the consequences of such reduction have been studied mainly in the context of nutrient utilization (Cahaner *et al.*, 1987; Ajang *et al.*, 1993; Leeson and Walsh, 2004a, b).

HEAT STRESS EFFECTS ON THE PERFORMANCE OF MODERN INDUSTRIAL BROILERS

Chickens, like all homeothermic animals, maintain a constant body temperature over a wide range of AT. In birds, heat loss is limited by the feather coverage and by the lack of sweat glands. The ability of animals to maintain BT within the normal range depends on a balance between internally produced heat and the rate of heat dissipation. The amount of internal heat produced by broilers depends on their BW and feed intake. Rate of heat dissipation depends on environmental factors, mainly AT, and on feather coverage. When the physiological and behavioural responses to high AT are inadequate, an elevation in BT occurs, causing a decrease in appetite and in GR. Consequently, the time needed to reach marketing body weight increases, leading to poorer feed conversion ratio (FCR) and lower overall efficiency of poultry meat production (Cahaner and Leenstra, 1992; Leenstra and Cahaner, 1992; Settar *et al.*, 1999). Moreover, hot conditions depress the yield and quality of broiler meat (Leenstra and Cahaner, 1992; Mitchell and Sandercock, 1995; Sandercock *et al.*, 2001), and may lead to PSE (pale, soft, exudative) meat (Barbut, 1997). Thus, high AT has been the main factor hindering broiler meat production in hot climates, especially in developing countries where farmers cannot afford costly artificial control of AT in broiler houses.

LIMITED SUCCESS OF SELECTION FOR HIGH MARKETING BODY WEIGHT UNDER HOT CONDITIONS

Breeding for adaptation to a specific stressful environment is the strategy of choice when genotype–environment (G×E) interaction affects economically important traits (Mathur and Horst, 1994). Such breeding may take place in a particular stressful location (localized breeding) or under induced stress. Commercial localized breeding under suboptimal hot conditions has been applied successfully in India (Jain, 2004). When compared under hot conditions, the imported broiler stocks were inferior to the locally bred stock. However, in absolute terms the latter performance was lower than the genetic potential of the imported broilers. Thus, it appears that standard broilers cannot be bred to exhibit high GR and high BW (in absolute terms) under hot conditions. So far, the latter has not been an important limitation in most hot-climate countries where customers traditionally prefer to buy live broilers with small body (about 1.5 kg), because heat hardly affects broilers up to that low BW. However, broilers that are produced for mechanical slaughtering and processing must have large BW at marketing and high yield of quality meat – the traits most depressed in high-GR broilers reared under hot conditions. Therefore, with the current trend to increase production of carcass parts and deboned meat catching up also in hot-climate countries, either for export or for local consumption, it will no longer be possible to avoid the negative effects of heat by marketing small-body broilers.

EFFECTS OF THE NAKED NECK GENE (*Na*) ON FEATHER COVERAGE AND HEAT TOLERANCE

Many studies had been conducted with the co-dominant ‘Naked neck’ (*Na*) gene, which is common in rural chickens in hot regions (Merat, 1986). This gene reduces feather coverage by 20% and 40% in heterozygous (*Na/na*) and homozygous (*Na/Na*) chickens, respectively (Crawford, 1976; Cahaner *et al.*, 1993; Yunis and Cahaner, 1999; Cahaner *et al.*, 2008). Merat (1986) suggested that the *Na* gene may improve heat tolerance. Under heat, naked-neck broilers exhibited greater sensible heat loss (Yahav *et al.*, 1998, 2005) and better thermoregulation (Eberhart and Washburn, 1993; Deeb and Cahaner, 1999), resulting in greater GR and meat yield than their fully feathered counterparts (Cahaner *et al.*, 1993; Yalcin *et al.*, 1997; Deeb and Cahaner, 2001). Yet naked-neck birds raised at 25°C were superior to their counterparts at hot conditions, suggesting that the 20% or 40% reduction in feather coverage provides only partial heat tolerance. Hence it was hypothesized that complete feather elimination may enhance heat tolerance of genetically fast-growing modern broilers (Cahaner *et al.*, 2003; Cahaner, 2008). The genetic and developmental mechanisms of naked neck have been revealed recently (Mou *et al.*, 2011), leading to a revived interest in these phenotypes and their contribution to heat tolerance in chickens.

THE SCALELESS GENE (*sc*)

Abbott and Asmundson (1957) reported a recessive mutation called 'Scaleless' that blocks feather formation in homozygous (*sc/sc*) embryos. They found the mutants in a flock of New Hampshire breed, which is much lighter and slow growing than modern meat-type chickens, hence they were not considered for practical purposes (Somes, 1990). In the 1970s, experimental featherless birds were derived from a cross between the scaleless mutant and commercial broilers of that time. In hot conditions, GR and carcass composition of these featherless birds were superior to those of their feathered counterparts (Somes and Johnson, 1982), but the effects were small because GR of the birds in this study was low, with a maximum of 30 g/day and average BW of about 1200 g at 8 weeks, compared with about 100 g/day in today's broilers that reach the same BW in about 4 weeks.

Development of a new line of featherless broilers was initiated in 2000 by crossing original (New Hampshire) scaleless mutants with contemporary industrial broilers, followed by a series of backcrossing and selection on BW (Cahaner and Deeb, 2004). The birds in this line were either normally feathered (+/*sc*, carriers of *sc* allele) or featherless (*sc/sc*), both with a genetic potential only slightly lower than that of contemporary industrial broilers. When compared with their feathered sibs (brothers and sisters with the same genetic background), the featherless broilers were exhibiting the net effects of being featherless under the trial's conditions.

WELFARE AND VIABILITY OF FEATHERLESS BROILERS VERSUS THEIR FEATHERED COUNTERPARTS

At an early stage of the development of this experimental line, featherless birds and their feathered sibs were exposed to heat waves in AT-controlled rooms

(Azoulay *et al.*, 2011). On day 47, the AT was gradually elevated from 30°C to 35°C for 2 days; consequently, BT elevated to 42.8°C in the feathered birds, and only to 41.4°C in the featherless birds. On day 53 (when BW averaged 1900 g), AT was abruptly elevated to 36°C, leading to lethal elevation of BT and death of 17 feathered birds (35%), whereas BT of the featherless birds remained at 41.4°C, and only one of 27 birds died. In a recent trial, after additional cycles of backcrossing that enhanced the potential GR of the experimental line, featherless broilers and their feathered sibs, as well as feathered commercial broilers, were kept together under constant hot conditions (32±1°C). When the birds were 41 days old (BW of about 1750 g), AT in one room increased unintentionally to 38°C for 5 h. Consequently, 20 of 28 commercial broilers died (71%), 30 of 72 feathered sibs died (42%), and only two of 100 (2%) featherless birds died (unpublished data). This event, and a similar one about 2 years later, demonstrated the association between potential GR and susceptibility to acute heat in standard (feathered) broilers, and proved the exceptional resistance to acute heat stress of the featherless birds, regardless of their genetic potential for GR. The results indicate that the welfare and livability of featherless broilers are not compromised under both acute as well as chronic hot conditions. The ability to maintain normal BT even under extreme AT is apparently the key to heat tolerance of the featherless broilers. Elevated BT under heat stress was shown to have a negative effect on GR, feed consumption and feed conversion in standard broilers (Cooper and Washburn, 1998). The results suggest that the superior GR and meat yield of featherless broilers under heat stress, compared with standard broilers, are due to their capacity to dissipate all the excessive internally produced heat and to maintain normal BT, and consequently normal feed consumption and GR.

Performance of featherless broilers versus feathered counterparts

Featherless broilers and their feathered sibs, with modern broilers as industry reference, were compared for performance traits under AT treatments (after brooding) of either constant 35°C (Hot-AT) or constant 25°C (Control-AT) (Azoulay *et al.*, 2011). All broilers were reared intermingled to 46 or 53 days at Control-AT and Hot-AT, respectively. Measured traits included BT, GR and weight of whole-body and carcass parts, breast meat, legs, wings and skin. At Hot-AT, only the featherless broilers maintained normal BT; their mean 46-day BW (2031 g) was significantly higher than at Control-AT, and it increased to 2400 g on day 53, much higher than the corresponding means of all feathered broilers (about 1700 g only). The featherless broilers had significantly higher breast meat yield (about 20% in both ATs), suggesting that the saved feather-building nutrients contributed to their higher breast meat yield. Skin weight was lower in the featherless broilers due to lack of feather follicles and low levels of cutaneous fat; with these features, the wings are leaner, hence supposedly of better quality (Azoulay *et al.*, 2011). The results confirmed that being featherless improves the performance of modern broilers in hot conditions and suggest that introduction of the featherless trait into modern stocks may facilitate highly efficient yet low-cost production of broiler meat in hot conditions (Cahaner *et al.*, 2010a, b).

Effects of being featherless on meat yield and quality in normal and hot conditions

Hot conditions reduce the feed intake as well as cardiovascular capacity in these broilers and consequently reduction in breast meat yield and its quality are often observed. The latter may lead to PSE Cpale, soft, exudative meat, possibly due to insufficient capillary support. With their heat tolerance, featherless broilers were expected to maintain high meat yield and quality in hot conditions. Accordingly, featherless broilers (*sc/sc*), their feathered sibs (+/*sc*) and contemporary broilers (+/+) were subjected to control AT (26°C) and hot AT (32°C) to test the hypothesis that lack of feathers contributes to higher breast muscle yield and better meat quality, especially under hot conditions, and that differences related to lack of feathers are related to cardiovascular capacity. In two similar trials, the superior genetic background of the contemporary broilers was manifested under control conditions; their mean BW was about 15% higher than the means of the featherless broilers and their feathered sibs. The hot conditions depressed BW of the two feathered groups by approximately 25%, with hardly any effect on featherless broiler BW. Breast meat yield (% of BW) in the featherless broilers was higher than in those with feathers, especially under the hot AT (Hadad *et al.*, 2014a). Furthermore, the featherless broilers were characterized by superior meat quality as indicated by lower drip loss, lower lightness and higher redness. The superior meat quality of the featherless broilers could be explained by their larger hearts and higher haematocrit values, suggesting superior cardiovascular capacity to supply oxygen and nutrients to the breast muscles (Hadad *et al.*, 2014a).

Another study was carried out to test the hypothesis that the advantage to the featherless broiler condition with respect to breast meat yield and quality is due to differences in muscle development during pre- and post-hatch periods. Broilers from the three genetic groups were reared under normal (26°C) and hot (32°C) conditions and slaughtered on day 29 and day 47 (Hadad *et al.*, 2014b). Evaluation of myofibre diameter (mean and distribution) and blood-vessel density in breast muscle sections sampled on these days revealed that the fluctuations in breast muscle yields of the different genetic groups under different temperature conditions and the better muscle growth of the featherless broilers were due to changes in muscle hypertrophy and vascularization (Hadad *et al.*, 2014b). In addition, the featherless broilers presented continuous satellite cell proliferation and a slower rate of differentiation compared with the feathered broilers in the immediate post-hatch period, suggesting a higher reserve of myogenic progeny cells, which would contribute to later muscle hypertrophy. In the embryos, breast muscle yield was higher for the featherless versus feathered counterparts between embryonic (E) days E15 and E20. This was manifested in a shift toward higher myofibre diameters in the featherless embryos on E18, and a higher number of myoblasts, which could be explained by higher insulin-like growth factor-I (IGF-I) levels in the muscle tissue and lower triiodothyronine (T3) levels in the plasma on E17. Together, the data showed the advantage of being featherless under hot conditions with regard to breast muscle growth and hypertrophy, and overall performance. Moreover, featherless embryos had increased breast muscle weight compared with their feathered counterparts, likely due to a higher proliferation rate of myoblasts and higher muscle hypertrophy (Hadad *et al.*, 2014b).

Nutrition of featherless versus feathered broilers under normal and hot conditions

Trials on the effects of dietary protein and energy content on performance of feathered versus featherless broilers were conducted under temperate (26°C) and hot (32°C) conditions. Commercial 3rd (days 17–31) and 4th (days 31–46) diets were used as Control. Experimental diets had lower contents (down to 80% of control diets) of protein or energy or both. Body weight gain and feed consumption were recorded until the end of the trial, when breast meat yield was determined (Tsur *et al.*, 2010). Under temperate conditions, lower protein and energy contents in the diluted diets reduced body weight and breast meat yield in the feathered broilers, but not in the featherless broilers. The featherless broilers have lower protein requirement, as could be expected because they do not need the amino acids used to build the feathers in standard broilers. With these lower requirements, being featherless improves also the economic FCR (cheaper feed), and reduces the environmental impacts of processing, by avoiding the plucking and dumping of the feathers.

Effects of stocking density on feathered versus featherless broilers under hot conditions

In tropical developing countries (e.g. Indonesia) where broiler producers cannot afford costly cooling and ventilation, production of relatively large and meaty broilers is based on modern stocks reared at low stocking density of about 7–8 birds/m^2. Trials were conducted to quantify the effects of stocking density under hot conditions on actual GR and meat yield and quality of feathered broilers versus featherless ones (Yadgari *et al.*, 2006). The feathered broilers were reared at densities in the range of 7–17 birds/m^2 whereas the featherless broilers were reared at densities in the range of 12–22 birds/m^2. The growth of the feathered broilers was depressed by higher stocking density; mean BW on day 44 decreased from 2.4 kg (7 birds/m^2) to 1.8 kg (17 birds/m^2). The growth of the featherless broilers was only marginally affected by stocking density, with mean BW of 2.4 kg (12 birds/m^2), 2.2 kg (17 birds/m^2) and 2.1 kg (22 birds/m^2); the latter resulted in total mass of 46 kg/m^2. The combined stress of heat and high stocking density reduced breast yield of modern feathered broilers to 15%, with pale meat (L*=50, a*=4) (where L* = lightness, a* = redness) and 4% drip loss. In the featherless broilers, breast yield was 19% in all stocking densities, with darker meat (L* = 44 and a* = 5) and less than 2% drip loss. Thus, in contrast to the negative association between genetic potential for rapid growth and high meat yield and quality of feathered broilers under heat (e.g. Mitchell and Sandercock, 1995), featherless broilers produced high yield of quality breast meat in hot conditions also at high stocking density (Cahaner *et al.*, 2010a,b).

PRACTICAL CONCLUSIONS

The results of many studies clearly indicate that modern featherless broilers cannot reach normal BW, as well as yield and quality of breast meat, under hot conditions. It appears that broiler meat production in hot regions and climates can be substantially improved by introducing the featherless gene into contemporary commercial broiler stocks. This has become more feasible since the detection of the *sc* mutation (Wells *et al.*, 2012) and the consequent development of a simple DNA test to identify carriers of the recessive *sc* mutation.

REFERENCES

Abbott, U.K., and Asmundson, V.S. (1957) Scaleless, an inherited ectodermal defect in domestic fowl. *Journal of Heredity* 48, 63–70.

Ajang, O.A., Prijono, S. and Smith, W.K. (1993) Effect of dietary protein content on growth and body composition of fast & slow feathering broiler chickens. *British Poultry Science* 34, 73–91.

Azoulay, Y., Druyan, S., Yadgary, L., Hadad, Y. and Cahaner, A. (2011) The viability and performance at hot conditions of featherless broilers vs. fully-feathered broilers. *Poultry Science* 90, 19–29.

Barbut, S. (1997) Problem of pale, soft, exudative meat in broiler chickens. *British Poultry Science,* 38, 355–358.

Cahaner, A. (2008) Breeding fast-growing, high-yield broilers for hot conditions. In: Daghir, N.J. (ed.) *Poultry Production in Hot Climates,* 2nd edn. CAB International, Wallingford, UK, pp. 30–47.

Cahaner, A. and Deeb, N. (2004) Breeding broilers for adaptability to hot conditions. In: *Proceedings of the 22nd World Poultry Congress*, Istanbul, Turkey.

Cahaner, A. and Leenstra, F. (1992) Effects of high temperature on growth and efficiency of male and female broilers from lines selected for high weight gain, favorable feed conversion, and high or low fat content. *Poultry Science* 71, 1237–1250.

Cahaner, A., Dunnington, E.A., Jones, D.E., Cherry, J.A. and Siegel, P.B. (1987) Evaluation of two commercial broiler male lines differing in efficiency of feed utilization. *Poultry Science* 66, 1101–1110.

Cahaner, A., Deeb, N. and Gutman, M. (1993) Effects of the plumage-reducing naked-neck (*Na*) gene on the performance of fast-growing broilers at normal and high ambient temperatures. *Poultry Science* 72, 767–775.

Cahaner, A., Druyan, S. and Deeb, N. (2003) Improving broiler meat production, especially in hot climates, by genes that reduce or eliminate feather coverage. *British Poultry Science* 44, 22–23.

Cahaner, A., Ajuh, J.A., Siegmund-Schultze, M., Azoulay, Y., Druyan, S. and Valle Zárate, A. (2008) Effects of the genetically reduced feather coverage in naked neck and featherless broilers on their performance under hot conditions. *Poultry Science* 87, 2517–2527.

Cahaner, A., Azoulay, Y., Tsur, N., Yadgary, L. and Hadad, Y. (2010a) Featherless broilers facilitate sustainable efficient meat production under hot conditions. In: *Procedings of the 13th European Poultry Conference*, Tours, France. Available at: http://www.wpsa.com/index.php/publications/wpsa-proceedings/2010/xiii-european-poultry-conference/2623-featherless-broilers-facilitate-sustainable-efficient-meat-production-under-hot-conditions/file (accessed 11 October 2018).

Cahaner, A., Tsur, N., Azoulay, Y., Yadgary, L. and Hadad, Y. (2010b) Featherless broilers may lower the costs and the environmental impact of poultry meat production under hot conditions. In: *Proceedings of the 9th World Congress on Genetic Application to Livestock Production*, Leipzig, Germany.

Cangar, O., Aerts, J.M., Buyse, J. and Berckmans, D. (2008) Quantification of the spatial distribution of surface temperatures of broilers. *Poultry Science* 87, 2493–2499.

Cooper, M.A. and Washburn, K.W. (1998) Relationship of body temperature to weight gain, feed consumption, and feed utilization in broilers under heat stress. *Poultry Science* 77, 237–242.

Crawford, R.D. (1976) Incomplete dominance of the gene for naked-neck on apteria width in domestic fowl. *Poultry Science* 56, 1683–1685.

Deeb, N. and Cahaner, A. (1999) The effect of naked-neck genotypes, ambient temperature, feeding status and their interactions on body temperature and performance of broilers. *Poultry Science* 78, 1341–1346.

Deeb, N. and Cahaner, A. (2001) Genotype-by-environment interaction with broiler genotypes differing in growth rate, 1. The effects of high ambient temperature and naked-neck genotype on stocks differing in genetic background. *Poultry Science* 80, 695–702.

Deeb, N., and Cahaner, A. (2002) Genotype-by-environment interaction with broiler genotypes differing in growth rate, 3. Growth rate, water consumption and meat yield of broiler progeny from weight-selected vs. non-selected parents under normal and high ambient temperatures. *Poultry Science* 81, 293–301.

Eberhart, D.E. and Washburn, K.W. (1993) Variation in body temperature response of naked neck and normally feathered chickens to heat stress. *Poultry Science* 72, 1385–1390.

Hadad Y., Halevy, O. and Cahaner, A. (2014a) Featherless and feathered broilers under control versus hot conditions. 1. Breast meat yield and quality. *Poultry Science* 93, 1067–1075.

Hadad Y., Cahaner, A. and Halevy, O. (2014b) Featherless and feathered broilers under control versus hot conditions. 2. Breast muscle development and growth in pre- and post-hatch periods. *Poultry Science* 93, 1076–1087.

Hanzl, C.J. and Somes, R.G. (1983) The effect of the naked neck gene, *Na*, on growth and carcass composition of broilers raised in two temperatures. *Poultry Science* 62, 934–941.

Havenstein, G.B., Ferket, P.R. and Qureshi, M.A. (2003a) Growth, livability, and feed conversion of 1957 vs. 2001 broilers when fed representative 1957 and 2001 broiler diets. *Poultry Science* 82, 1500–1508.

Havenstein, G.B., Ferket, P.R. and Qureshi, M.A. (2003b) Carcass composition and yield of 1957 vs. 2001 broilers when fed representative 1957 and 2001 broiler diets. *Poultry Science* 82, 1509–1518.

Jain, G.L. (2004) Breeding for special needs of developing countries in collaboration with international companies. In: *Proceedings of the 22nd World Poultry Congress*, Istanbul, Turkey. World's Poultry Science Association, Beekbergen, Netherlands.

Leenstra, F. and Cahaner, A. (1992) Effects of low, normal, and high temperatures on slaughter yield of broilers from lines selected for high weight gain, favorable feed conversion, and high or low fat content. *Poultry Science* 71, 1994–2006.

Leeson, S. and Walsh, T. (2004a) Feathering in commercial poultry. I. Feather growth and composition. *World Poultry Science Journal* 60, 42–51.

Leeson, S. and Walsh, T. (2004b) Feathering in commercial poultry. II. Factors influencing feather growth and feather loss. *World Poultry Science Journal* 60, 52–63.

Mathur, P.K. and Horst, P. (1994) Genotype by environment interactions in laying hens based on relationship between breeding values of sires in temperate and tropical environments. *Poultry Science* 73, 1777–1784.

Merat, P. (1986) Potential usefulness of the Na (Naked Neck) gene in poultry production. *World Poultry Science Journal* 42, 124–142.

Mitchell, M.A. and Sandercock, D.A. (1995) Increased hyperthermia induced skeletal muscle damage in fast growing broiler chickens? *Poultry Science* 74(Suppl.1), 74.

Mou, C., Pitel, F., Gourichon, D., Vignoles, F., Tzika, A. *et al.* (2011) Cryptic patterning of avian skin confers a developmental facility for loss of neck feathering. *PLOS Biology* 9, 1–13.

Sandercock, D.A., Mitchell, M.A. and MacLeod, M.G. (1995) Metabolic heat production in fast and slow growing broiler chickens during acute heat stress. *British Poultry Science* 36, 868.

Sandercock, D.A., Hunter, R.R., Nute, G.R. and Mitchell, M.A. (2001) Acute heat stress induced alterations in blood acid base status and skeletal muscle membrane in broiler chickens at two ages, implications for meat quality. *Poultry Science* 80, 418–425.

Settar, P., Yalcin, S., Turkmut, L., Ozkan, S. and Cahaner, A. (1999) Season by genotype interaction related to broiler growth rate and heat tolerance. *Poultry Science* 78, 1353–1358.

Somes, R.G. (1990) Mutations and major variants of plumage and skin in chickens. In: Crawford, R.D. (ed.) *Poultry Breeding and Genetics*. Elsevier, Amsterdam, The Netherlands, pp. 169–208.

Somes, R.G., and Johnson, S. (1982) The effect of the scaleless gene, *sc*, on growth performance and carcass composition of broilers. *Poultry Science* 61, 414–423.

Tsur, N., Uni, Z. and Cahaner, A. (2010) Effects of dietary protein and energy content on performance of feathered vs featherless broilers in hot conditions. In: *Proceedings of the 13th European Poultry Conference*, Tours, France.

Wells, K., Hadad, Y., Ben-Avraham, D., Hillel, J., Cahaner, A. and Headon, D.J. (2012) Genome-wide SNP scan of pooled DNA reveals nonsense mutation in FGF20 in the Scaleless line of featherless chickens. *BMC Genomics* 13, 257–266.

Yadgari, L., Kinereich, R., Druyan, S. and Cahaner, A. (2006) The effects of stocking density under hot conditions on growth, meat yield and meat quality of featherless and feathered broilers. *World's Poultry Science Journal* 62(Suppl.), 603–604.

Yahav, S., Straschnow, A., Plavnik, I. and Hurwitz, S. (1997) Blood system responses of chickens to changes in environmental temperature. *Poultry Science* 76, 627–633.

Yahav, S., Luger, D., Cahaner, A., Dotan, M., Rusal, M. and Hurwitz, S. (1998) Thermoregulation in naked-neck chickens subjected to different ambient temperatures. *British Poultry Science* 39, 133–138.

Yahav, S., Shinder, D., Tanny, J. and Cohen, S. (2005) Sensible heat loss, the broiler's paradox. *World's Poultry Science Journal* 61, 419–434.

Yalcin, S., Testik, A., Ozkan, S., Settar, P., Celen, F. and Cahaner, A. (1997) Performance of naked-neck and normal broilers in hot, warm, and temperate climates. *Poultry Science* 76, 930–937.

Yunis, R. and Cahaner, A. (1999) The effects of the naked-neck (*Na*) and frizzle (*F*) genes on growth and meat yield of broilers, and their interactions with ambient temperatures and potential growth rate. *Poultry Science* 78,1347–1352.

CHAPTER 10
The Genetics of Contact Dermatitis in Poultry

Dagmar N.R.G. Kapell*
Aviagen Ltd, Newbridge, Scotland

ABSTRACT

The prevalence of contact dermatitis traits is an important consideration in modern poultry production, as part of the general focus on leg health and welfare traits. Contact dermatitis is seen as a lesion or discolouration of the skin, potentially accompanied by inflammation or necrosis. Various scoring systems have been developed, often relating ordinal scores to the proportional area affected. Environmental factors have a significant effect on its prevalence, but studies have shown that genetic variation exists for foot pad dermatitis (FPD) in chickens and turkeys and for hock burn in chickens. This review shows genetic parameters for contact dermatitis traits in contemporary chicken and turkey populations in the Aviagen breeding programmes, and their genetic correlations with production traits. FPD is recorded in all Aviagen breeding programmes, with hock burn additionally recorded in the Aviagen chicken breeding programmes. All traits are scored at commercially relevant ages on a four or five point scale (depending on trait/species) through visual inspection by a trained team of scorers. Heritabilities for FPD in chickens range from 21% to 32% and for hock burn from 9% to 23%. Genetic correlations with body weight are generally favourable (FPD) or moderately unfavourable (hock burn). Heritabilities for FPD in turkeys range from 5% to 16%, with low to moderately unfavourable genetic correlations with body weight. Genetic selection to improve contact dermatitis has been incorporated effectively for chickens and turkeys in commercial breeding programmes. The differences in heritability for FPD between the species may be due to fundamental differences of the expression of contact dermatitis, despite similar phenotypes. However, in both species genetic correlations with a production trait were only low to moderately unfavourable or even favourable. In broad breeding goals, where the focus lies simultaneously on welfare traits and production traits,

*dkapell@aviagen.com

progress can be achieved simultaneously despite potentially antagonistic correlations.

INTRODUCTION

Contact dermatitis is an ulceration of the skin in chickens and turkeys, usually seen as a lesion or discolouration of the skin, potentially accompanied by inflammation or necrosis (Martland, 1984; Greene *et al.*, 1985; Mayne, 2005). Environmental factors such as litter quality and stocking density have a significant effect on the prevalence (Shepherd and Fairchild, 2010). Various scoring systems have been developed over the years, generally relating ordinal scores to the proportion of surface area affected by lesions or discolouration (e.g. Kjaer *et al.*, 2006; Hocking *et al.*, 2008; Ask, 2010). Several studies have shown that genetic variation exists for foot pad dermatitis (FPD) in both chickens and turkeys and for hock burn (HB) in chickens (e.g. Kjaer *et al.*, 2006; Ask, 2010; Quinton *et al.*, 2011; Kapell *et al.*, 2012a, 2012b, 2017,). Contact dermatitis traits are included in both chicken and turkey breeding goals to reduce the genetic predisposition of birds to develop these conditions and as a part of a balanced selection to improve biological performance, health and welfare.

TRAIT DESCRIPTION AND PHENOTYPIC DISTRIBUTIONS

The data for the analysis originates from the ongoing recording of a broad range of leg health traits within the Aviagen chicken and turkey breeding programmes, which includes contact dermatitis traits, but also others related to skeletal strength and walking ability. The trait FPD has been recorded in all Aviagen chicken and turkey breeding programmes since 2006, while HB has been recorded in the Aviagen chicken breeding programmes since 1990.

In chickens, FPD is recorded on a three-point scale, according to the extent to which the lesions cover the pad of the foot (Kapell *et al.*, 2012a). The scores range from 0 (no lesions) through 1 (up to 50% covered) to 2 (more than 50% covered). The trait HB is scored on a four-point scale, ranging from 0 (no lesions) through 1 (up to 25% covered) and 2 (up to 50% covered) to 3 (more than 50% covered) (Kapell *et al.*, 2012b). Both traits are scored at 5–6 weeks, depending on line. In turkeys, FPD is scored on an extended scale of five points, and, like in chickens, depends on the extent to which the foot pad is covered by lesions. The scores in turkeys range from 0 (no lesions) through 1 (up to 25% covered), 2 (up to 50% covered) and 3 (up to 75% covered) to 4 (up to 100% covered) (Kapell *et al.*, 2017). The trait is scored at 18 weeks.

Scoring of FPD and HB is done through visual inspection of both feet and hocks by a trained team of evaluators who are regularly assessed for consistency of scoring, both within and between evaluators. A stringent selection approach is used whereby the worst score of the two feet determines the final score for the individual bird. A more detailed description of the scores, including figures, has been reported previously for FPD in chickens (Kapell *et al.*, 2012a), HB in chickens (Kapell *et al.*, 2012b) and FPD in turkeys (Kapell *et al.*, 2017).

Both in chickens and turkeys there is considerable variation between genetic lines in the proportion of birds per score. In chickens the large majority of the birds (circa 60%) have a score of 0, meaning no FPD is seen (Fig. 10.1) for a range of different elite commercial lines. While there is an overall pattern of similarity in FPD scores for all lines, there are still considerable differences between them. Similarly, a large majority of birds (circa 80%) across the four lines showed no HB lesions (Fig. 10.2). Lesions covering more than 50% of the hock were not seen at all. Interestingly, the chicken line with the higher proportion of birds

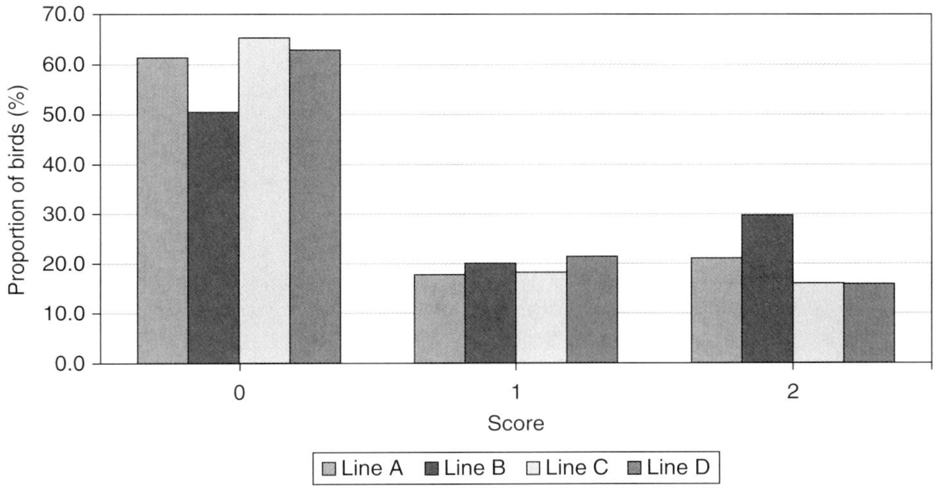

Fig. 10.1. Distribution of foot pad dermatitis (FPD) scores by category in chicken lines A to D.

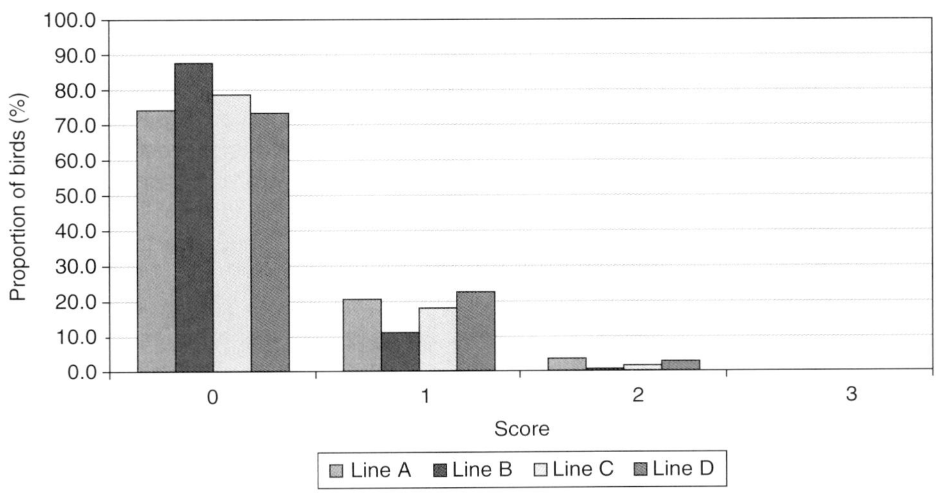

Fig. 10.2. Distribution of hock burn (HB) scores by category in chicken lines A to D.

scoring 1 or 2 for FPD had the highest proportion of birds with no HB (score 0), suggesting an absence of a strong correlation between FPD and HB in chickens.

The distribution of birds across FPD scores is more even in turkeys (Kapell *et al.*, 2017) compared with chickens. Around 40–50% of the birds have a score of 2, meaning that between 25% and 50% of the foot pad is covered by lesions; 15–30% of the birds had a score of 1 or 3 and the remaining birds a score 0 or 4.

GENETIC ANALYSIS

Variance components were estimated per line with a multivariate animal model using restricted maximum likelihood (REML) as implemented in the variance component estimation (VCE) software package (Groeneveld *et al.*, 2008). For this analysis FPD and HB were transformed to a 100–200 scale. The linear models included a fixed effect accounting for the interaction between the hatch week, pen, contributing mating group and sex of the individual, as well as the random permanent environmental effect of the dam and the additive genetic effect of the animal. The models included body weight (BWT), FPD and HB (chickens only) in two environments. These two environments are a high bio-secure pedigree (P) environment, where breeding programme selection candidates are recorded and selected under optimal conditions, and a non-bio-secure sib-test (S) environment, where siblings of selection candidates are tested under broader commercial-like conditions (Kapell *et al.*, 2012a, 2017). In the following section, traits recorded in the sib-test environment are denoted by an 'S' at the start, i.e. SBWT, SFPD and SHB.

Heritabilities for FPD in chickens were on average 28% in the P environment and 24% in the S environment, but with some variation between lines, especially in the P environment where it ranged from 21% to 32% (Fig. 10.3). The heritability of HB was lower, on average 14% in the P environment (with a range from 9% to 23%), and as low as 1% in the S environment. The latter was likely due to the low prevalence of HB in this environment. At the phenotypic level the correlations within trait between the two environments were low at 0.20 or less for FPD and HB. However, genetic correlations within trait were much higher between environments (Fig. 10.4). For FPD the correlation was consistent between lines, averaging 0.71 with a range of 0.68–0.73 across lines. For HB a much wider range of 0.14–0.67 was observed, which may be due in part to the low heritability seen in the S environment. Genetic correlations with production traits, such as BWT, were generally low. For FPD they were on average –0.13 in the P environment and –0.01 in the S environment, which indicates no genetic antagonism between BWT and FPD (Fig. 10.5). For HB the genetic correlations were slightly antagonistic at on average 0.34 in the P environment and 0.35 in the S environment.

In turkeys the heritabilities for FPD were lower, averaging 11% in the P environment and 10% in the S environment (Fig. 10.6), with less variation between lines (ranges from 5% to 16% and 9% to 11% in the P and S environment,

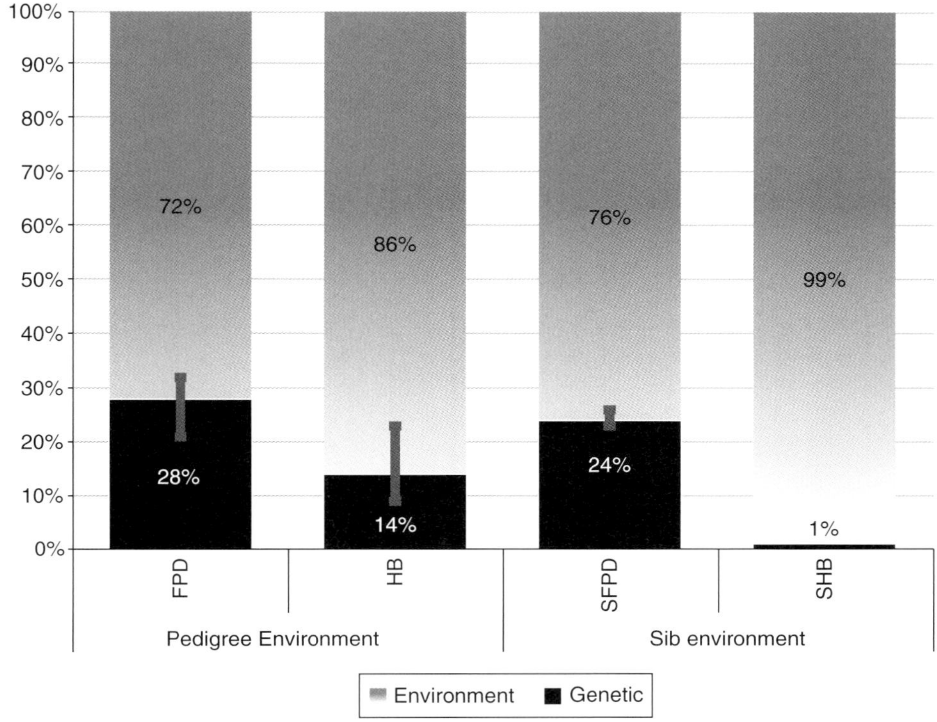

Fig. 10.3. Range of the proportion of variation attributable to genetic or environmental factors for foot pad dermatitis (FPD) and hock burn (HB) in chickens.

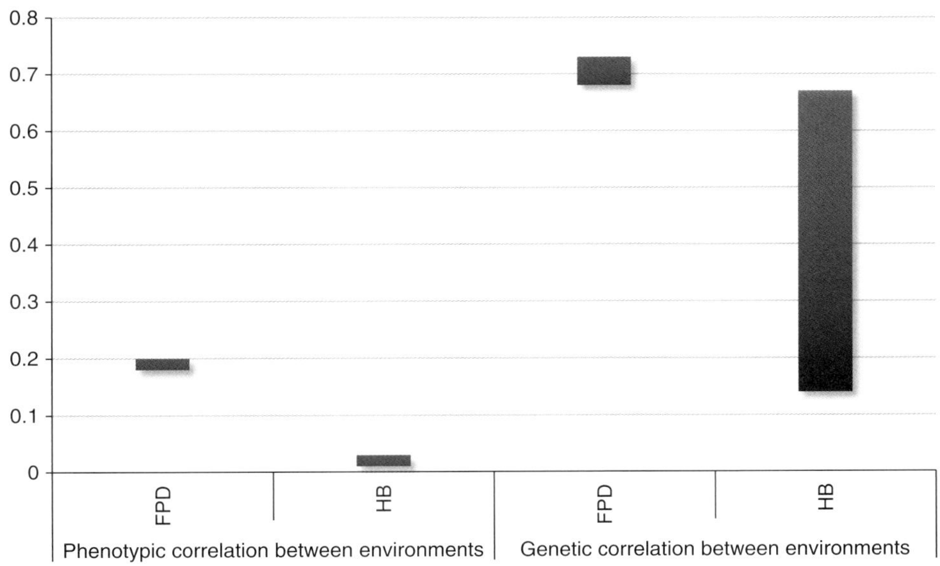

Fig. 10.4. Range of phenotypic and genetic correlations within trait between different environments for foot pad dermatitis (FPD) and hock burn (HB) in chickens.

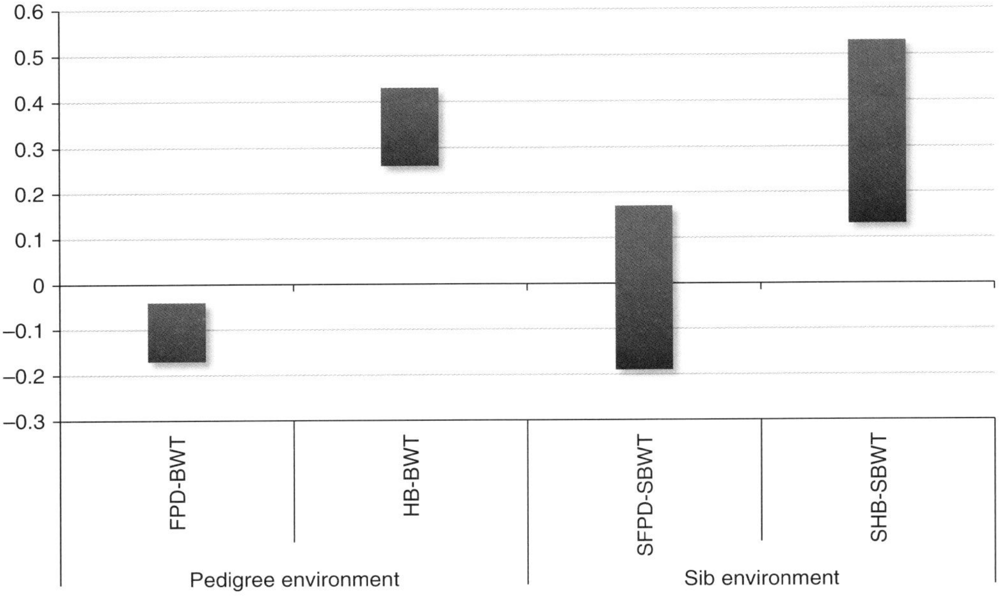

Fig. 10.5. Range of genetic correlations of foot pad dermatitis (FPD) or hock burn (HB) with body weight (BWT) in chickens in different environments.

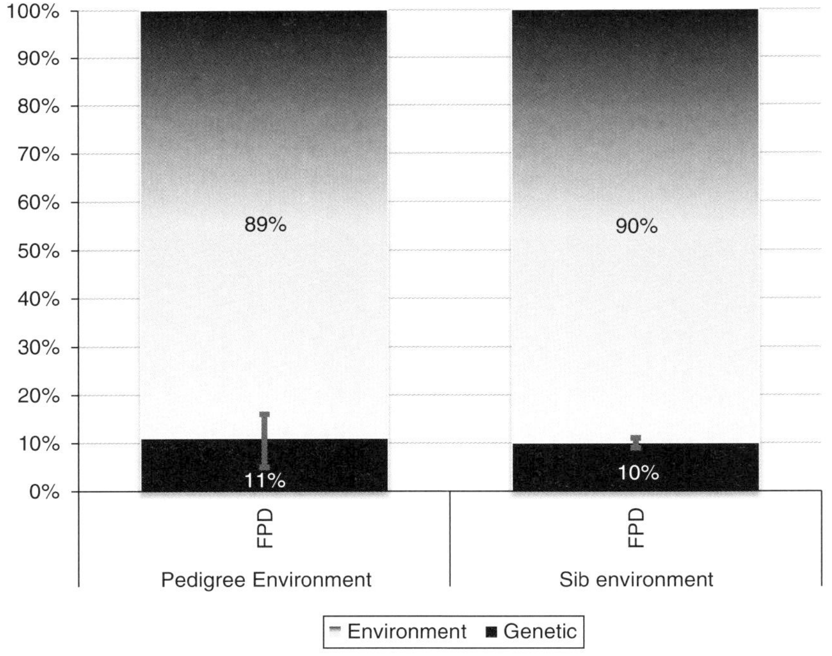

Fig. 10.6. Range of the proportion of variation attributable to genetic or environmental factors for foot pad dermatitis (FPD) in turkeys.

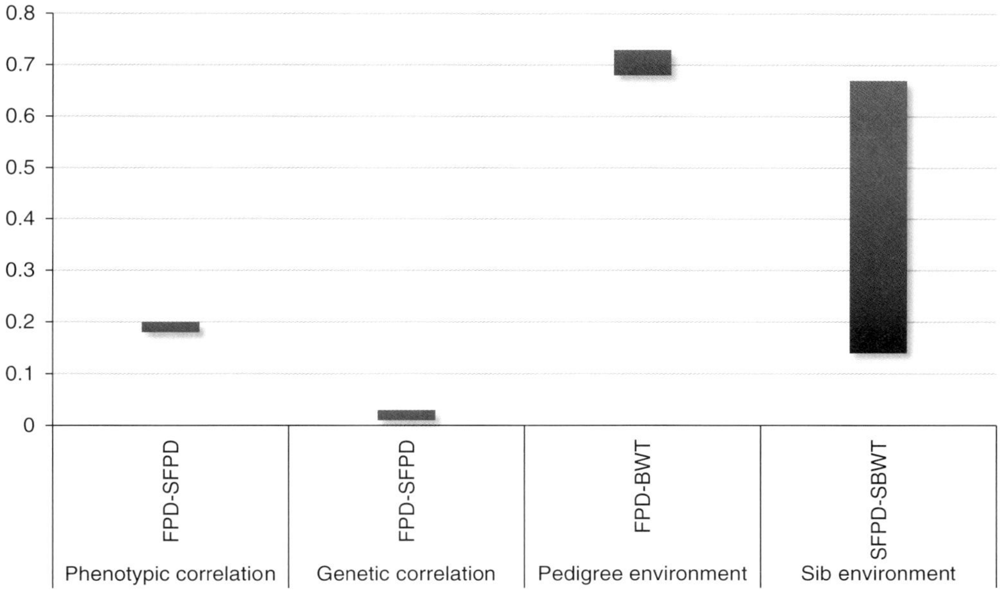

Fig. 10.7. Range of correlations within the trait foot pad dermatitis (FPD) between different environments, as well as between FPD and body weight (BWT), in turkeys.

respectively) (Fig. 10.7). Despite low phenotypic correlations (on average 0.10), genetic correlations were high at on average 0.85. Notwithstanding the small range for the heritabilities for FPD, the range of the genetic correlations with BWT in the P environment was wide, ranging from as low as 0.12 up to 0.55. In the S environment the correlations between BWT and FPD were less strong, from 0.10 to 0.24.

SIMULTANEOUS IMPROVEMENT OF TRAITS WITH ANTAGONISTIC RELATIONSHIP

Despite low to moderately antagonistic relationships between traits, a multi-trait breeding goal allows for genetic progress to be achieved both within an environment and across environments. While correlations between production and welfare related traits may be unfavourable, with correlations less than 1 (i.e. the correlation is less than perfect) there will always be selection candidates available that provide genetic progress on traits. Figure 10.8 shows an example of the estimated breeding values (EBVs) for a group of chicken selection candidates, where the correlation between BWT and HB is unfavourable. Figure 10.9 shows a similar example for turkeys, where the genetic correlation between SFPD and SBWT is around 0. These figures illustrate how a set of birds in one quadrant (highlighted in dark grey) can have desirable breeding values for both traits simultaneously. By selecting such birds to breed the next generation, steady progress can be and has been achieved in a range of traits, despite somewhat unfavourable correlations (Fig. 10.10 chickens and Fig. 10.11 turkeys) (Kapell *et al.*, 2012a, b, 2017).

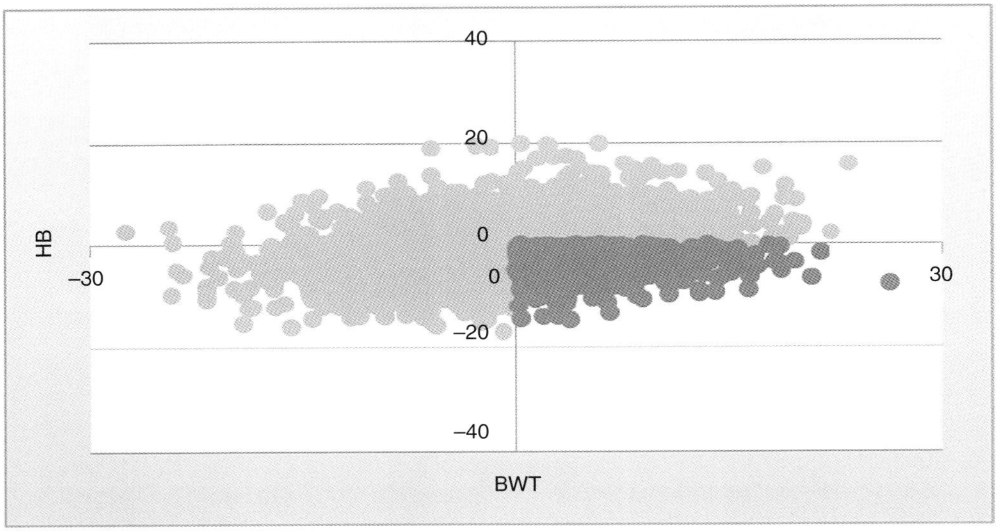

Fig. 10.8. Range of estimated breeding values (EBVs) for hock burn (HB) versus body weight (BWT) in the pedigree environment for a group of selection candidates in chickens. The dark grey quadrant shows birds with a favourable EBV for both traits.

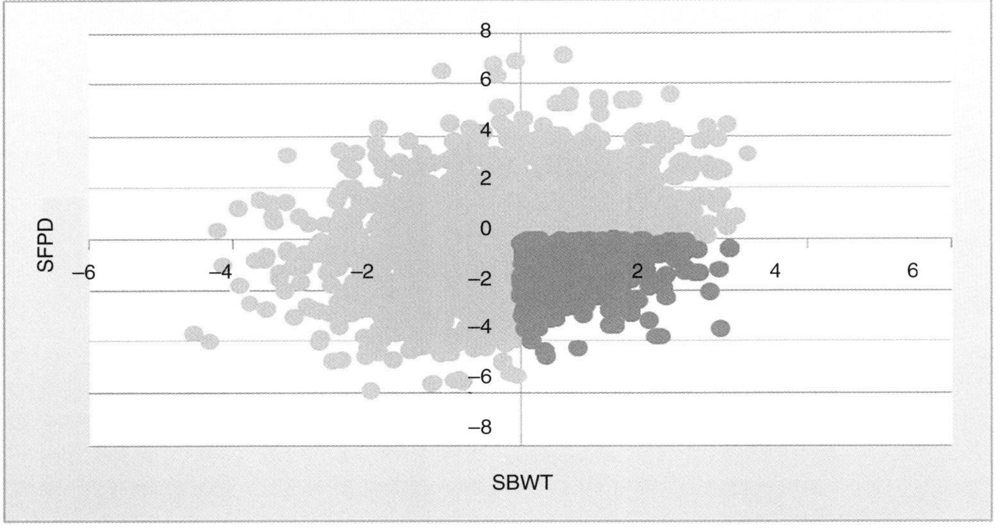

Fig. 10.9. Range of estimated breeding values (EBVs) for foot pad dermatitis (FPD) versus body weight (BWT) in the sib(S)-test environment for a group of selection candidates in turkeys. The dark grey quadrant shows birds with a favourable EBV for both traits.

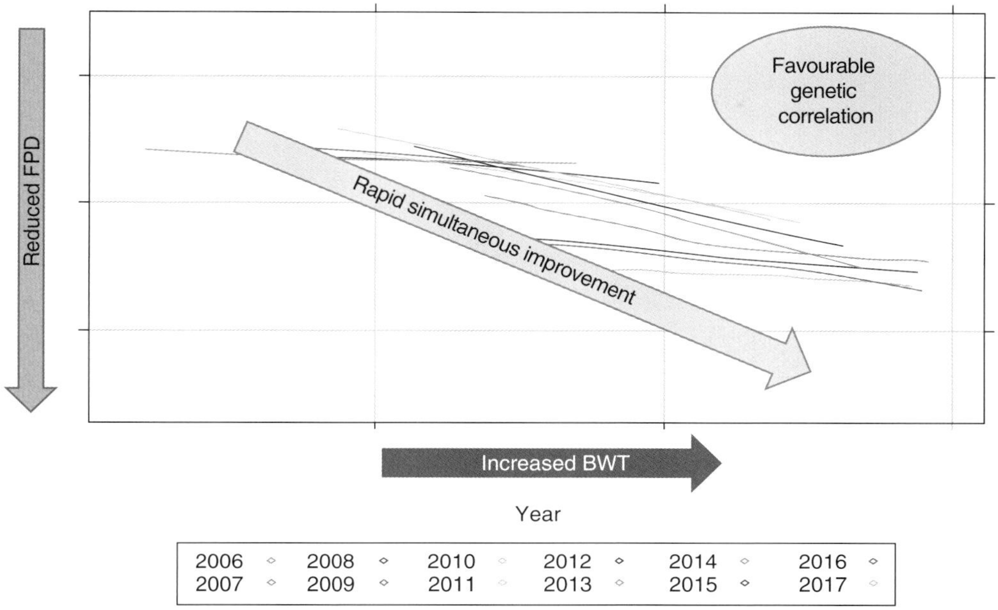

Fig. 10.10. Correlation between the estimated breeding value (EBV) for foot pad dermatitis (FPD) and the EBV for body weight (BWT) within the year from 2006 to 2017 for chickens, showing the progress made on both traits in the presence of favourable genetic correlations.

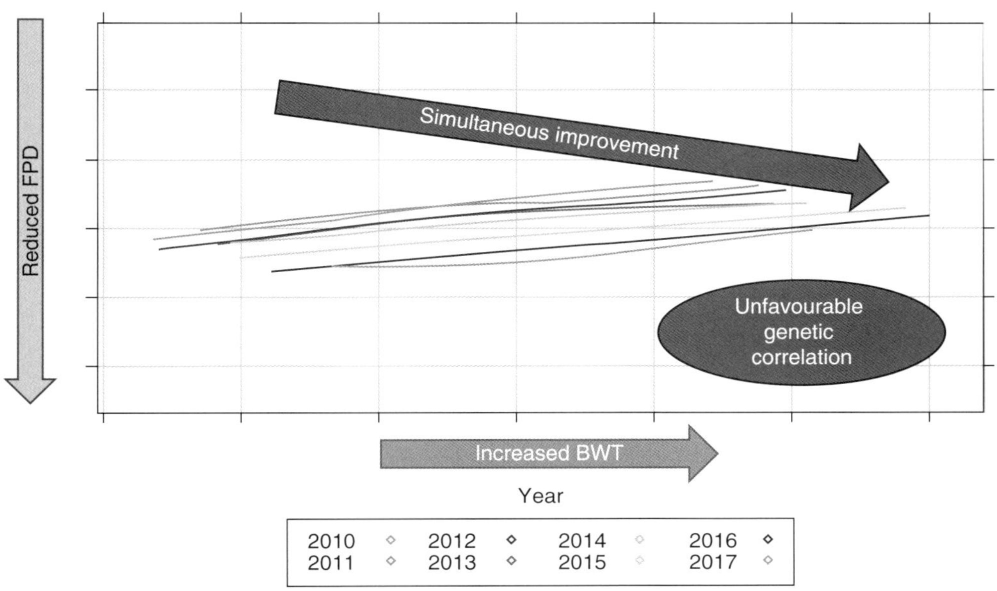

Fig. 10.11. Correlation between the estimated breeding value (EBV) for foot pad dermatitis (FPD) and the EBV for body weight (BWT) within the year from 2010 to 2017 for turkeys, showing the progress made on both traits in the presence of unfavourable genetic correlations.

CONCLUSION

Genetic selection to improve contact dermatitis has been incorporated effectively for both chickens and turkeys in commercial breeding programmes. The differences in heritability for FPD between the two species may be due to fundamental differences of the expression of contact dermatitis between species, despite similar phenotypes. However, in both species genetic correlations with a production trait were only low to moderately unfavourable or even favourable. In broad breeding goals, where the focus lies simultaneously on welfare traits and production traits, our experience shows that progress can be and has been achieved simultaneously despite potentially antagonistic correlations.

REFERENCES

Ask, B. (2010) Genetic variation of contact dermatitis in broilers. *Poultry Science* 89, 866–875.

Greene, J.A., McCracken, R.M. and Evans, R.T. (1985) A contact dermatitis of broilers – clinical and pathological findings. *Avian Pathology* 14, 23–23.

Groeneveld, E., Kovač, M. and Mielenz, N. (2008) *VCE User's Guide and Reference Manual.* Version 6.0. Institute of Farm Animal Genetics, Neustadt, Germany.

Hocking, P.M., Mayne, R.K., Else, R.W., French, N.A. and Gatcliffe, J. (2008) Standard European footpad dermatitis scoring system for use in turkey processing plants. *World's Poultry Science Journal* 64, 323–328.

Kapell, D.N.R.G., Hill, W.G., Neeteson, A.M., McAdam, J., Koerhuis, A.N.M. and Avendaño, S. (2012a) Genetic parameters of foot-pad dermatitis and body weight in purebred broiler lines in 2 contrasting environments. *Poultry Science* 91, 565–574.

Kapell, D.N.R.G., Hill, W.G., Neeteson, A.M., McAdam, J., Koerhuis, A.N.M. and Avendaño, S. (2012b) Twenty-five years of selection for improved leg health in purebred broiler lines and underlying genetic parameters. *Poultry Science* 91, 3032–3043.

Kapell, D.N.R.G., Hocking, P.M., Glover, P.K., Kremer, V.D. and Avendaño, S. (2017) Genetic basis of leg health and its relationship with body weight in purebred turkey lines. *Poultry Science* 96, 1553–1562.

Kjaer, J.B., Su, G., Nielsen, B.L. and Sørensen, P. (2006) Foot pad dermatitis and hock burn in broiler chickens and degree of inheritance. *Poultry Science* 85, 1342–1348.

Martland, M.F. (1984) Wet litter as a cause of plantar pododermatitis, leading to foot ulceration and lameness in fattening turkeys. *Avian Pathology* 13, 241–241.

Mayne, R.K. (2005) A review of the aetiology and possible causative factors of foot pad dermatitis in growing turkeys and broilers. *World's Poultry Science Journal* 61, 256–267.

Quinton, C.D., Wood, B.J. and Miller, S.P. (2011) Genetic analysis of survival and fitness in turkeys with multiple-trait animal models. *Poultry Science* 90, 2479–2486.

Shepherd, E.M. and Fairchild, B.D. (2010) Footpad dermatitis in poultry. *Poultry Science* 89, 2043–2051.

Part IV
Nutrition and Management

CHAPTER 11
Effects of Nutritional Interventions on Feathering of Poultry – a Review

Rick A. van Emous* **and Marinus M. van Krimpen**
Wageningen Livestock Research, Wageningen, The Netherlands

ABSTRACT

Feather cover of chickens can be influenced by many factors, including direct or indirect nutritional factors. Direct dietary factor effects are levels of protein/amino acids, vitamins, minerals and mycotoxins. Indirect nutritional factors will impact feather cover through their effects on feather pecking behaviour. Since feathers contain 89–97% protein, the supply of dietary amino acids plays a critical role in feather development. Particularly in the juvenile phase of broilers and breeders, low dietary crude protein intake can negatively affect feather quality. Especially the sulfur-containing amino acids methionine and cystine are indicated as necessary for the synthesis of feather keratin. Dietary deficiencies of these amino acids have been shown to result in rough feathering, as indicated by body feathers sticking out from the body, or malformed cover feathers on the wings of young and older birds. Deficiencies of vitamin E and selenium might lead to depigmentation and shorter shafts of wing feathers, whereas deficiencies of other vitamins can lead to slower feather development and swollen tip of down feathers. Mineral (zinc, tin, vanadium, chromium, nickel) deficiencies could result in delayed feather development, frayed feathers (zinc) and blisters on the shafts. Mycotoxins in the feed have been shown to cause sparse covering of feathers and sticking out of feathers from the body. In an indirect way, nutritional aspects can also affect feather cover due to feather pecking in chickens. There is strong evidence that a (very) low crude protein content (<13%) of the diet increases injurious pecking in laying hens. On the other hand, a low energy content of the diet might decrease mortality of laying hens because the dilution of the diet increases eating time. Adding roughage (maize silage, barley silage or carrots) to the daily feed decreases injurious pecking behaviour and increases plumage condition of laying hens. Adding tryptophan to layer diets reduces

*rick.vanemous@wur.nl

incidences of feather pecking, because this AA contributes to serotonin turnover in the brain, which is largely related to bird behaviour. Addition of (coarse) insoluble non-starch proteins has been shown to increase gizzard weight and its contents and to prolong mean retention time in the foregut, which is an indicator for higher levels of satiety and a reduced motivation to peck. This chapter gives an overview of the direct and indirect relationships between the effects of nutritional interventions on feathering of poultry.

INTRODUCTION

Feathers are very important for chickens because of their role in thermoregulation and in prevention of skin damage by other chickens and equipment. It is well known that feed consumption increases when feather cover of layers decreases (Peguri and Coon, 1993; Glatz, 2001). Poor feather cover in broilers can lead to skin damage, with negative effects on carcass quality (Urdaneta-Rincon and Leeson, 2004). In breeders, feathers play an important role to protect broiler breeders from skin damage caused by sharp objects in the house and from damage during rough mating behaviour of the male (De Jong *et al.*, 2009). The above-mentioned effects of poor feather cover have a major impact on the profitability of the layer, broiler and breeder industries.

Feather growth and development in chickens can be affected by a wide range of different factors such as housing, temperature, health status and management (Deschutter and Leeson, 1986). Besides these factors, nutrition plays a major role in feather growth and development and can be divided into direct and indirect factors (Van Krimpen *et al.*, 2005). Direct dietary effects are levels of protein/amino acids (AA), vitamins, minerals and mycotoxins, whereas feather pecking behaviour, and the consequential impact on feather cover, might be an indirect nutritional effect. The objective of this chapter is to provide an overview of the direct and indirect nutritional effects on feathering of poultry.

FEATHER COMPOSITION

Feathers comprise 89–97% protein (Fisher *et al.*, 1981; Stilborn *et al.*, 1997) whereas the protein content of keratin is 85–90% (Harrap and Woods, 1964). This keratin is a durable fibrous protein (Kemp and Rogers, 1972) that is virtually resistant to degradation by most of the enzymes (Leeson and Walsh, 2004a). The major AA involved in the synthesis of feather keratin is the sulfur AA, cystine (Wheeler and Latshaw, 1981), which suggests a high dietary requirement of this amino acid (Leeson and Walsh, 2004a). The other sulfur AA, methionine, is involved through its conversion to cystine, which occurs both in the liver and in the feather follicle (Champe and Maurice, 1984). No consistent and recent data about AA composition of feathers is available in the literature (Fisher *et al.*, 1981; Stilborn *et al.*, 1997). It was shown by Fisher *et al.* (1981) that the AA composition of feathers of broilers was relatively stable during the growing period, with small increases of threonine, valine and leucine and decreases in methionine content. A consistent AA content of feathers was confirmed by Stilborn *et al.* (1997) (Fig. 11.1). From Fig. 11.1 it is clear that the amino acids leucine, cystine, arginine and valine are important building blocks of feathers.

Compared with the AA composition of tissue (total carcass) (Stilborn *et al.*, 2010), feathers contain more cystine (7.5% versus 1.0%), phenylalanine (4.7% versus 3.8%), valine (6.2% versus 4.7%) and threonine (4.8% versus 4.1%) (Fig. 11.2). In contrast, feathers contain less lysine (2.0% versus 6.9%), histidine (0.7% versus 2.5%) and methionine (0.7% versus 2.2%) than tissue.

FEATHER DEVELOPMENT AND MOULTING

During the transition period from chick to mature bird (rearing), a series of moulting periods to a mature feather cover have been identified (Leeson and Walsh, 2004a). All follicles are already formed during the embryo state and after hatch the number of follicles is fixed. Conditions during incubation might affect feather development (Merat and Coquerelle, 1991). The latter authors reported impaired feather growth in broiler embryos when eggs were hatched at 38.6°C compared with 37°C (control) in the second week of the hatching period. After hatch, chicks are covered with a dense coat of down feathers and the wing feathers are the earliest feathers (first moult). Usually, in broilers, the second moult starts at 4–5 weeks of age, which is also the last moult (Leeson and Walsh, 2004a). The

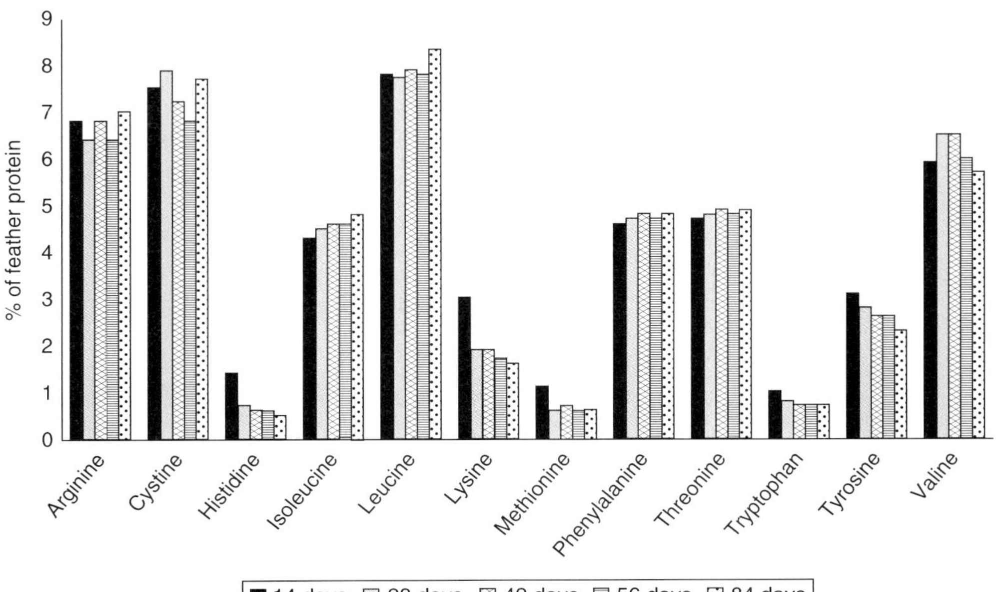

Fig. 11.1. Development of amino acids composition of feathers in growing broilers while ageing (adapted from Stilborn *et al.*, 1997).

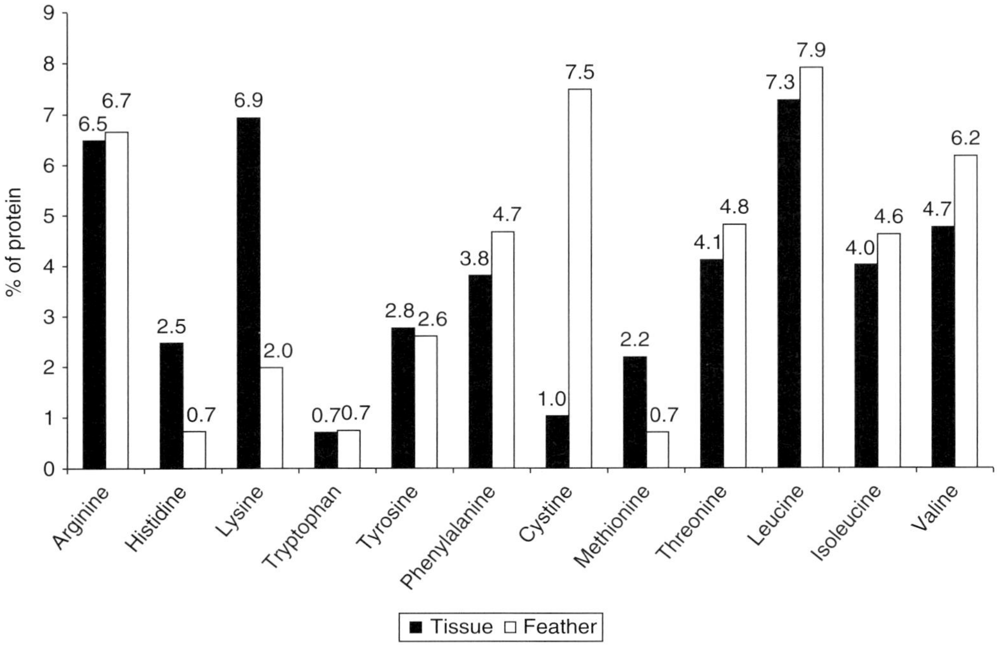

Fig. 11.2. Comparison of amino acids composition of tissues and feathers in growing broilers (adapted from Stilborn *et al.*, 1997, 2010).

second moult in layers and broiler breeders falls roughly between 2 and 6 weeks of age, whereas the third moulting period is between 10 and 16 weeks of age (Moran, 1981; Aviagen, 2013). However, besides the different moulting periods identified, during the juvenile stage of life feathers are continuously shed and re-synthesized on a lower level until a mature feather cover is formed (Deschutter and Leeson, 1986). Under acute stress birds can instantaneously shed some of their feathers, which might represent an evolutionary-evolved mechanism to escape from predators (Ostmann *et al.*, 1963). Feather cover varies considerably during lifetime and decreases during the laying period of breeders and layers (M.M. van Krimpen, Wageningen, 2017).

After the first laying period, flocks are sometimes subjected to a so-called 'forced' moulting period prior to a new production cycle period (Leeson and Walsh, 2004a). After such forced moulting, layer flocks often have significantly improved feather cover, though feather cover does not usually recover fully to the quality at the beginning of the first laying period (LaBrash and Scheideler, 2005).

During the past two decades, more and more so-called 'fault bars' or 'stress lines' have been mentioned for different bird species (Jovani and Blas, 2004; Strochlic and Romero, 2008; Jovani and Rohwer, 2017). This phenomenon is defined as feather malformations, generated during feather growth, resulting in a translucent line perpendicular to the rachis (King and Murphy, 1984; Jovani and Rohwer, 2017). They appear as transparent cross-bands approximately 1 mm wide in the feather flag (Fig. 11.3). The keratin deposition during growth of the feather is disturbed in this part of the feather, causing a weakness in the structure which can, in the worst case, result in broken feathers (e.g. Newton, 2010). Fault bars are induced by psychological stress due to malnutrition, age, sex, disease, corticosterone and habitat (Jovani and Rohwer, 2017). That fault bars in broiler breeders can be caused by acute stress has been studied by Arrazola *et al.* (2017), who applied three different unpredictable stress situations (physical restriction during 20 min, crowding during 2 h, or delayed feeding of 2–3 h) in breeders between 3 and 6 weeks of age. They concluded that the development of fault bars was affected by the type of feather (wing rather than tail feathers), that acute stress induced the development of moderate fault bars in wing feathers and that the total number of fault bars in wing feathers increased in individual susceptible birds.

DIRECT AND INDIRECT DIETARY EFFECTS RELATED TO FEATHER COVER

Feather cover development can be affected by a wide range of different factors such as housing, temperature, health status, management, and nutrition (Deschutter and Leeson, 1986). Nutrition can have direct and indirect effects on feather growth and development (Van Krimpen *et al.*, 2005). Direct dietary effects are levels of protein (AA), vitamins, minerals, and mycotoxins, whereas the effect of nutrition on feather pecking might be considered as an indirect effect on feather cover.

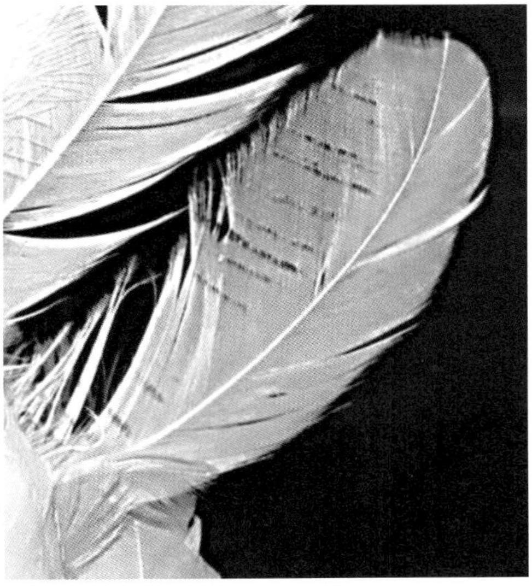

Fig. 11.3. Fault bars in a broiler breeder tail feather (photograph courtesy of A. Arrazola, 2017).

Direct effects

Crude protein

Broiler chickens until 6 weeks of age require about 10% of their daily dietary protein intake for feather formation (Stilborn *et al.*, 1997; Hancock *et al.*, 1995). Due to the high level of crude protein (CP) and AA in feathers (Stilborn *et al.*, 1997) a sufficient supply of these nutrients via the diets is of great importance. The importance of CP (and AA) had been mentioned by Twining *et al.* (1976), who carried out two broiler studies with different dietary CP (and AA) levels. In the first experiment, broilers received a 4.5% (absolute) lower CP diet between 0 and 49 days of age followed by a 3.5% lower CP diet during the finisher phase. In the second experiment, birds received the same starter diet between 0 and 28 days of age and a 4.5% and 3.5% lower CP diet in the finisher diet (28–49 days of age) and finisher diet (49–59 days of age), respectively. In both experiments they found, in general, consistently more feathers on the litter and a lower feather cover score at the end of the growing cycle when birds were fed the higher CP diets. From these results, the authors concluded that feather growth and moulting of feathers was positively affected by the higher CP levels. The effect of CP on feather cover in broilers was confirmed by Urdaneta-Rincon and Leeson (2004), who observed in a study with 21-day-old broilers that a dietary CP increase from 170g/kg to 250g/kg resulted in an increased feather weight from 6.0g to 9.3g per bird and an increased feather nitrogen gain from 0.95g to 1.15g. An increase to 290g CP/kg, however, did not result in a further increase of feather weight or feather nitrogen gain. Comparable results of dietary CP level on feather growth and feather length were found in a study with young turkeys (Wylie *et al.*, 2003). A large male and small traditional line were fed four different diets with 180g, 220g, 260g and 300g CP/kg . The feather weight in the 180g/kg birds amounted 18% less for the large male and 24% less for the small traditional line as compared with the 300g/kg birds. Feather length in tail, back and wings decreased linearly with decreasing CP level, but an inconsistent effect was found for the cranial region of the breast. Feather length decreased from 26mm to 19mm in the traditional line compared with an increase from 14mm to 25mm in male-line turkeys.

Leeson and Walsh (2004b) postulated that a CP deficiency had a negative effect on feather development. When birds younger than 10 to 15 days of age were fed diets with less than 16% CP, invariably poorly feathered chicks were observed. This situation sometimes occurs in breeder pullets and it seems that CP level plays an important role in this phenomenon and cannot be easily solved by adding high levels of free amino acids to the diets (Leeson and Walsh, 2004b). This means that there is a certain requirement of crude protein or that knowledge on specific AA for an optimum feather cover development for breeder pullets is lacking (Leeson and Walsh, 2004b).

The sensitivity to low CP (and AA) levels in breeder pullets at young age was observed by Van Emous *et al.* (2014, 2015). During two experiments, pullets were fed a high (standard) or low balanced CP diet (both CP and important AAs were decreased in the same amount). During the starter (2–6 weeks of age), grower (6–15 weeks of age) and pre-breeder phase (15–22 weeks of age), pullets were fed diets containing 17.3%, 14.3% and 15.0% CP (high CP diets) or 14.7%, 12.4% and 13.0% CP (low CP diets). In the first experiment, a worse feather cover was observed at 6 and 11 weeks of age when pullets were fed the low CP diet (Van Emous *et al.*, 2014). This difference, however, diminished from 11 weeks of age onwards. In the second experiment, feather coverage was inferior for the low CP diet during the entire rearing period (Van Emous *et al.*, 2015) (Fig. 11.4). It was suggested by Van Emous (2015) that the CP and AA levels of the diets in the studies here were critical or deficient, in particular those AA needed for feather growth and development. This suggestion was underlined by the malformed cover feathers on the wings in the second study, which might be an indication of an AA deficiency. Moran (1984) had already showed that marginal dietary deficiencies of sulfur-containing AAs resulted in abnormal feathering.

Data of the first study were used to analyse the relationships between the feather score and the total CP intake at different phases during the rearing period (Fig. 11.5). Feather score decreased linearly with increasing CP intake during 2–6 weeks of age (Fig. 11.5, panel A; $P<0.001$), whereas no significant relationship was found later in life (Fig. 11.5, panel B; $P=0.182$). Thus, total CP

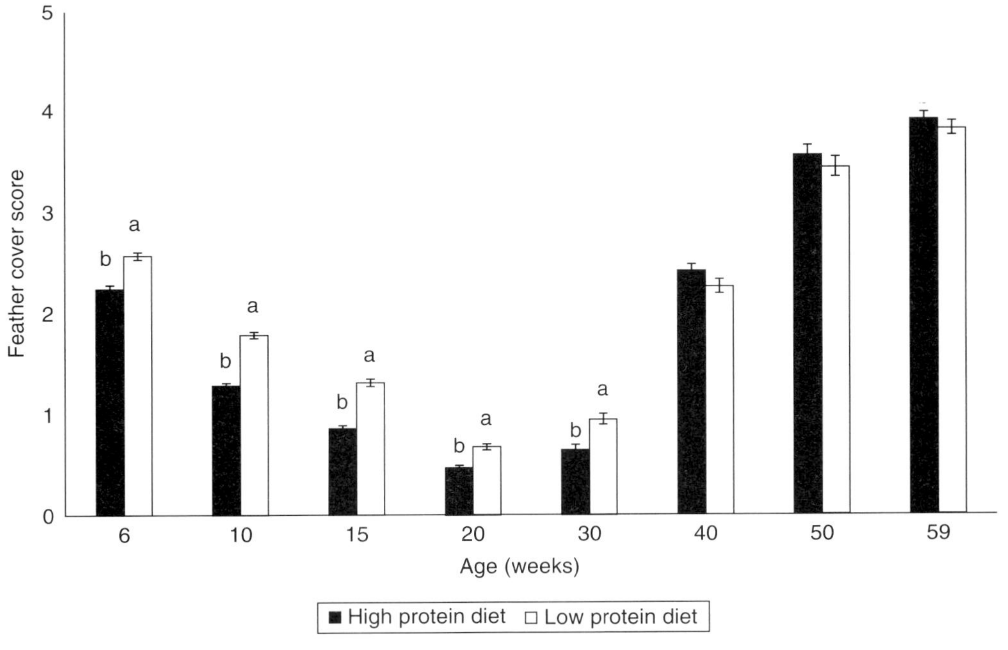

Fig. 11.4. Feather cover score (mean ± SEM) from 6 to 59 weeks of age for broiler breeder pullets reared on a high or low protein diet (Van Emous, 2015). [a,b]Different letters indicate significant differences among treatments ($P<0.05$) within age. Feather cover was scored from 0 (intact) to 5 (bald) for each of seven different body parts and averaged to a total feather cover score per bird (Bilcik and Keeling, 1999).

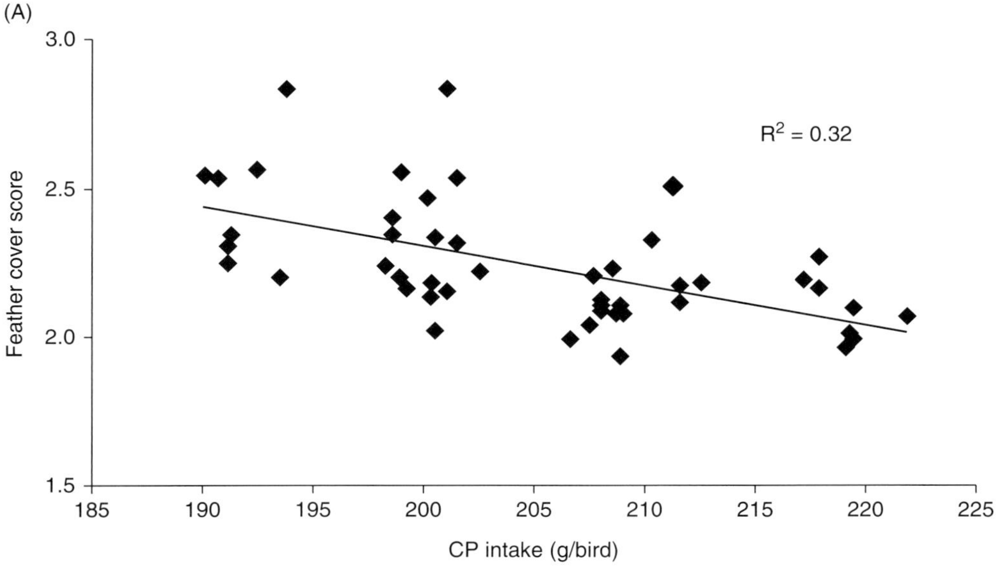

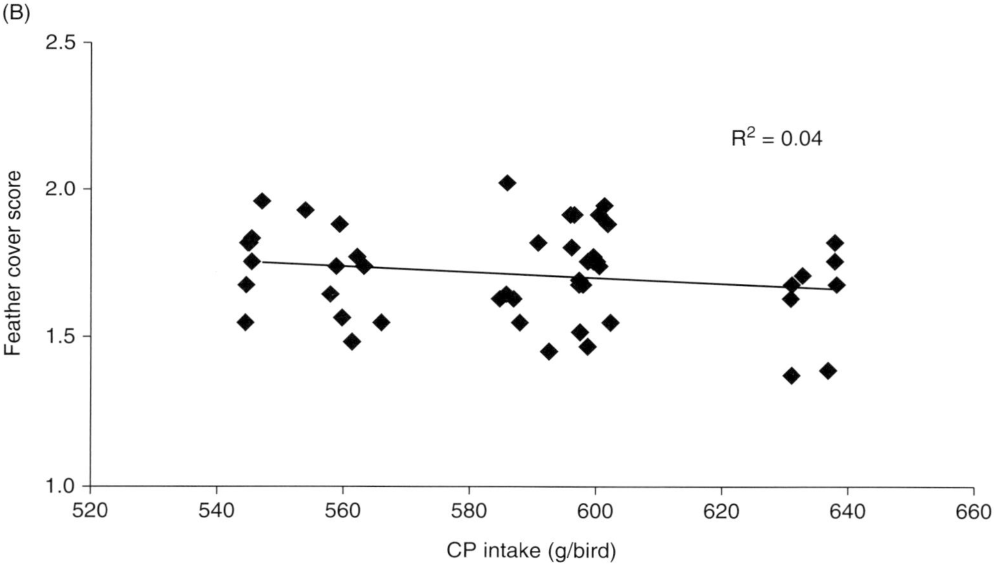

Fig. 11.5. Relationship between the total crude protein (CP) intake (g/bird) between 2 to 6 weeks of age (starter 2 diet; panel A) or between 6 to 15 weeks of age (grower diet; panel B) and feather cover scores at 6 weeks of age (panel A) or at 16 weeks of age (panel B). Points represent individual pens (Van Emous, 2015).

(and AA) intake is a critical factor in development of feather cover during rearing until at least 6 weeks of age, whereas in later life this relationship is less pronounced.

The breeder company Aviagen performed a study with Ross 708 broiler breeders to improve the feather cover during the laying period (L.B. Linares, personal communication). They applied a diet with 10% higher (relative) CP and AA levels during the entire laying period, and compared this diet with a standard diet with CP and AA levels recommended by the breeder company. Furthermore, they applied a diet with reduced (between 2% and 18% relative) CP and AA levels. No effect was found for the +10% CP/AA diet; however, the 2–18% lower CP/AA diet deteriorated the feather cover from 40 weeks onwards.

Lysine

Adding lysine to a low CP diet, such that the consumption of lysine increased from 485 mg to 587 mg per hen per day, improved plumage condition of laying hens considerably (Al Bustany and Elwinger, 1987b). In this dose–response trial, in which the total lysine content varied from 5.6 g/kg to 9.4 g/kg (resulting in increased CP levels), no further improvement of plumage condition was found from a lysine level of 8.2 g/kg onwards.

The previously mentioned study of Urdaneta-Rincon and Leeson (2004) was set up as a 4×3 factorial design with four different CP levels (170 g, 210 g , 250 g or 290 g CP/kg) and three different lysine levels. The 210 g, 250 g and 290 g CP/kg levels each contained either 0.86%, 1.34% or 1.46% lysine, whereas the 170 g CP/kg diet contained either 0.86%, 1.22% or 1.34% lysine. They concluded that dietary lysine levels from 0.86% to 1.46% did not affect feather-weight, feather nitrogen gain, or feather:body weight ratio in male chicks between 0 and 21 days of age.

Methionine and cystine

For the development of the most dominant protein of feathers (keratin), the sulfur-containing AAs (methionine and cystine) are of a great importance (Wheeler and Latshaw, 1981). Of these, cystine is the most important component of keratin (Fisher *et al.*, 1981; Stilborn *et al.*, 1997), while methionine is involved through its conversion to cystine (Champe and Maurice, 1984). It is in close agreement with the AA composition of feathers as observed by Stillborn *et al.* (1997), who found that feathers contained more cystine (7.5%) and only 0.7% methionine, which is an indication of a difference in importance between methionine and cystine. The effect of different levels of methionine and cystine on feather weight development in broilers was evaluated by Moran (1981), who found that an increased methionine level in a finisher diet (+0.5 g/kg or +1.0 g/kg) did not affect feather weight of broilers. On the other hand, a higher cystine level (between +0.5 g/kg and +1.8 g/kg) increased feather weight by 3% and 5% for males and females, respectively. In research by Kalinowski *et al.* (2003) with fast- and slow-feathering broilers, the optimal methionine level did not differ between fast- and slow-feathering broilers: for each type of birds the optimum amounted to 5 g/kg. For cystine, a substantial difference was found: the optimum cystine level amounted to 3.9 g/kg for slow-feathering and 4.4 g/kg for fast-feathering bids. These results further strengthen the notion that cystine is more important in the development of feathers in broilers than methionine. Methionine and cystine also have an effect on the texture of feathers. Tsiagbe *et al.* (1987) found stronger feathers when 0.20% cystine was supplemented to a basal diet containing 0.37% cystine with 0.35% methionine. Remarkably, adding a large dose of methionine (+1.45%) to a basal diet resulted in much softer feathers. It was postulated that these effects were caused by the content of bound sulfide.

Other amino acids

As previously shown, the sulfur-containing AAs (especially cystine) are the most important ones for feather development. However, several studies have suggested that other AAs are also important (Anderson and Warnick, 1967; Robel, 1977; Penz *et al.*, 1984; Farran and Thomas, 1992; Wylie *et al.*, 2003). Typical symptoms of AA deficiency are a spoon-like appearance of the primary and secondary feathers. Sanders *et al.* (1950) postulated that this was caused by the retention of an abnormally long sheath that covers the proximal end of the feather shaft. Another observation is the loss of their smooth appearance due to the absence of a normal interlocking between the barbules and barbs (Anderson and Warnick, 1967). Abnormal curling of the feathers away from the body is another sign of AA deficiency (Robel, 1977). These signs of abnormalities in feather development are reported in combination with diets deficient in arginine, valine, leucine, isoleucine, tryptophan, phenylalanine and tyrosine. In a study by Farran and Thomas (1992) chicks were fed a diet deficient in valine but with sufficient levels of leucine and isoleucine. They observed feather abnormalities as described previously. Therefore these authors concluded that a deficiency of valine alone had a higher negative impact on feather development compared with a deficiency of all branch-chain amino acids. Comparable feather abnormalities were found by Penz *et al.* (1984) when birds were fed high levels of leucine. They analysed the AA content of the diets for deficiencies of valine, isoleucine and cystine. Adding extra valine or isoleucine to the diet solved the problem of feather abnormalities.

Wylie *et al.* (2003) conducted an experiment with young turkeys (2–6 weeks of age) and added arginine, valine, methionine and tyrosine separately to a common basal ration (18% CP) to increase the CP to the level of the control diet (26% CP). The basal diet with added tyrosine resulted in a lower feather weight, whereas adding valine had no effect. Adding arginine or methionine to the basal diet resulted in a significantly higher feather weight similar to that of the control diet. They concluded that arginine and methionine were essential for feather growth whereas tyrosine and valine had no effect on feather cover.

Vitamins and minerals

Besides the effects of crude protein and amino acids, vitamins and minerals also play an important role in feather development (Leeson and Walsh, 2004b). Impaired feather development was observed by Supplee (1966) when turkey chicks were fed diets with low levels of vitamin E and selenium. Adding organic selenium to a broiler diet between 21 to 42 days of age, instead of sodium selenium (0.2 ppm), resulted in an increased development of feather cover (Edens *et al.*, 2001). Diets deficient in pyridoxine (Daghir and Balloun, 1963), pantothenic acid, folic acid, biotin or nicotinic acid (Taylor, 1967) showed more or less comparable negative effects on the quality of the feathers. Leeson and Summers (1997) observed very characteristic signs of swollen tips in down feathers in embryos and chicks due to a deficiency of riboflavin. The effects of single vitamins on the feather development in broilers were investigated by Summers *et al.* (1978), who found delayed feather development and primaries with barbs and barbules on only the distal part of the feather, though these effects were not characteristic for specific vitamins.

Deficiencies of trace minerals (zinc, tin, vanadium, chromium and nickel) resulted in delayed feather development and cover (Scott *et al.*, 1959; Baker and Molitoris, 1975). Supplee *et al.* (1958) were probably the first who found the importance of zinc for normal feather development of growing pullets. Scott *et al.* (1959) suggested that pheasant diets needed to be supplemented with zinc to prevent poor feather cover. Diets lacking in zinc results in frayed feathers, especially in the fast-growing primaries and secondaries (Sunde, 1972).

Mycotoxins

As well as CP levels, AAs and deficiencies of vitamins and minerals, dietary mycotoxins can affect feather cover (Leeson and Walsh, 2004b). Wyatt *et al.* (1975) found that birds fed T-2 toxin (produced by *Fusarium* spp.) showed a poor feather cover, which was probably caused by the alteration of the metabolism of certain nutrients involved in feather development. Typical for this mycotoxin was that feathers of the whole body were affected, whereas deficiencies of vitamins or AA seemed to adversely affect specific parts of the body. Problems with feather cover occurred at levels as low as 4–16 ppm T-2 toxin and were dose-dependent.

Indirect effects

Besides the direct effects of nutritional interventions on feather cover, indirect effects of nutrition – via mechanisms of feather pecking behaviour – are important. Feather pecking can be caused by many factors, such as management, rearing, health status and housing system. It is widely accepted that nutrition is another factor in this phenomenon.

Energy

It is suggested that feather pecking behaviour is influenced by the energy content of the diet (Van Krimpen *et al.*, 2005). In an experiment with layer diets with different energy levels (10.7, 11.2, 11.7 and 12.2 MJ/kg) several effects were found (Elwinger, 1981). Lower energy contents were associated with higher feed intakes, lower energy intakes, a tendency to lower mortality and a lower (i.e. better) feather cover score. This finding was confirmed by Van der Lee *et al.* (2001), who fed hens a low-density diet (11.05 MJ/kg) which resulted in better feather cover without effects on production performance, as compared with hens fed a standard diet (11.55 MJ/kg). In both experiments, feed intake was higher for the low-energy diets, which resulted in more time spent on feeding and less time remaining for stereotypic feather pecking behaviour (Van Krimpen *et al.*, 2005). This is in agreement with the research of Savory (1980), who fed male Japanese quail diets diluted with 40% cellulose or a standard (undiluted) diet. Birds receiving the diluted diets showed an approximately 40% higher feed intake, spent more time on feeding, and showed a longer meal length and a shorter inter-meal interval length and had more meals per day.

Crude protein

Seven decades ago, it was shown that feeding protein-deficient diets increased the risk of feather pecking and cannibalism in birds. Schaible *et al.* (1947) observed a lower incidence of feather pecking and cannibalism in laying pullets between 0 to 8 weeks of age when protein supplements (e.g. casein, gelatine, liver meal, blood meal) were added to a basal diet low in CP (135 g/kg). Ambrosen and Petersen (1997) conducted a study with seven different layer strains and found that a low protein diet (111 g/kg) without the addition of free amino acids resulted in almost 18.0% mortality due to cannibalism, compared with 2.5% mortality when layers were fed a diet of 193 g CP/kg. At first, this finding seems to contradict the work of Al Bustany and Elwinger (1987a), who found no effect on mortality of diets with CP contents of 124–176 g/kg (experiment 1) or 134–177 g/kg (experiment 2). This can be explained by the fact that significant effects of CP level on mortality were only found for levels of 126 g/kg and lower by Ambrosen and Petersen (1997), whereas Al Bustany and Elwinger (1987a) only used CP levels above 124 g/kg. Furthermore, in the second experiment of Al Bustany and Elwinger (1987a), a treatment group receiving 120 g CP/kg was excluded from the experiment because of high mortality due to cannibalism. In a previous experiment, Al Bustany and Elwinger (1986) had found no effects on feather cover and mortality of diets with CP levels of 124, 150 and 176 g/kg.

Amino acids

Comparison of a low versus a high CP and AA diet for organic laying hens (135 g CP/kg, 5.9 g Lys/kg and 5.1 g M + C/kg versus 169 g CP/kg, 8.7 g Lys/kg and 6.7 g M + C/kg) showed an inferior feather cover and a higher incidence of injuries of the comb and rear body parts due to pecking with diets low in CP and AA (Elwinger *et al.*, 2002). In contrast, no effect was found of a low (4.2 g/kg) versus a high (8.2 g/kg) level of methionine + cysteine in organic diets on feather cover of laying hens (Kjaer and Sørensen, 2002). For 4-week-old cockerels, feeding dietary levels of arginine at 6.9% or 3.9% of the total protein increased the level of cannibalism from 0 to 21% (Sirén, 1963).

A higher level of tryptophan (2.6–22.6 g/kg) in the diets of growing bantams resulted in a lower incidence of pecking damage (Savory, 1998; Savory *et al.*, 1999). It was suggested that this was probably caused by the lower level of severe feather pecking behaviour. This was confirmed by Van Hierden *et al.* (2004), who fed a diet to young chickens with a very high (21.0 g/kg) versus a standard (1.6 g/kg) tryptophan level. Tryptophan is known as a precursor for serotonin synthesis (5-HT) and chickens from a high feather-pecking line displayed lower 5-HT turnover levels in response to acute stress than chickens from a low feather-pecking line (Van Hierden *et al.*, 2002). Higher dietary tryptophan stimulates serotonergic neurotransmission, resulting in a higher turnover of tryptophan to 5-HT in the brain (Van Hierden *et al.*, 2004).

Feed form

It is well known that the physical form of the diet, e.g. mash, crumble or pellet, and the distribution of particle size in mash diets, can affect feather pecking behaviour, possibly due to differences in time spent on feeding (Van Krimpen *et al.*, 2005). Laying hens fed a coarse-ground meal (33–55% of particles > 2 mm) showed more feather pecking than hens fed a fine-ground meal (0–13% of particles > 2 mm) (Walser and Pfirter, 2001). A significant interaction was shown between feed form (mash or pellet) and foraging material (with or without long straw) (Aerni *et al.*, 2000). High rates of feather pecking and pronounced feather damage were only found in laying hens housed without straw and fed with pellets, indicating that laying hens (especially when fed pellets) should be provided with an adequate amount of foraging material. Laying hens with access to foraging material also had a lower ratio of heterophil to lymphocyte and an increased immune response to immunization than those without access to such materials, indicating lower stress in these birds (El Lethey *et al.*, 2000).

Roughage

It has been suggested by several authors that supplementing roughage to birds results in less feather pecking (Hoffmeyer, 1969; Köhler *et al.*, 2001; Steenfeldt *et al.*, 2001, 2007). Feeding young pheasants (between 5 and 10 weeks of age) cut green clover and branches with green leaves as roughage resulted in less feather pecking as compared with controls (Hoffmeyer, 1969). Supplementing carrots or maize silage to laying hens between 20 and 54 weeks of age resulted, at 24 weeks of age, in less gentle and severe feather pecking as compared with the control group and hens fed barley–pea silage (Steenfeldt *et al.*, 2001). At 53 weeks of age comparable tendencies of effects, though not significant, on behaviour were observed. Laying hens fed maize silage and barley–pea silage had the best feather cover at 53 weeks of age. In a second study, laying hens received, besides a standard diet, maize silage, barley–pea silage and carrots (Steenfeldt *et al.*, 2007). Egg production was significantly higher for the hens receiving carrots or maize silage as compared with hens fed barley–pea silage. Feeding all three types of supplement resulted in decreased damaging pecking in general (to feathers as well as skin/cloaca), reduced severe feather pecking behaviour and improved quality of the plumage at 54 weeks of age.

Non-starch polysaccharides

The effect of dietary energy dilution and non-starch polysaccharides (NSPs) concentration (oat hulls as NSP source) on eating behaviour and feather damage was studied by Van Krimpen (2008). In this study, an increased gizzard weight (and content) and a prolonged mean retention time in the foregut were found –

an indicator for a higher level of satiety. Furthermore, more feeding behaviour was found, as indicated by a longer eating time and a lower eating rate. Therefore, Van Krimpen (2008) concluded that enhancing feeding-related behaviour and satiety by dietary manipulation are successful strategies in preventing feather pecking behaviour, as long as this behaviour has not yet developed at an earlier stage.

SUMMARY AND CONCLUSION

The feather cover of chickens can be influenced by many factors, including direct and indirect nutritional factors. Direct dietary factors include: levels of protein/amino acids, vitamins and minerals; and presence of mycotoxins. Indirect dietary factors are mediated through the mechanisms of feather pecking behaviour. The available literature suggests that a sufficient supply of crude protein and more specifically the amino acids cystine (either directly or mediated through methionine), valine and arginine plays an important role in feather development. Dietary deficiencies of many amino acids may result in feather abnormalities. Deficiencies of the vitamin selenium can lead to depigmentation and shorter shafts of wing feathers and to slower feather development. Deficiencies in minerals (zinc, tin, vanadium, chromium, nickel) can result in delayed feather development, frayed feathers and blisters on the shaft. Mycotoxins in the feed can cause sparse covering of feathers and feathers protruding from the body. There is strong evidence that a (very) low crude protein content (<13%) stimulates injurious pecking in laying hens. A low energy content of the diet reduces pecking-related mortality in laying hens by means of dilution of the diet and prolonged eating time. Adding roughage (maize silage, barley silage or carrots) to the feed reduces injurious pecking behaviour and positively affects plumage condition of layers. Adding high levels of tryptophan to layer diets results in less feather pecking through its contribution to serotonin turnover. Addition of (coarse) insoluble NSP increases gizzard weight and its contents and increases retention time in the foregut, which is an indicator for a higher level of satiety and a reduced motivation to peck. In conclusion, providing nutritionally balanced and NSP-enriched feed is important to obtain and maintain good feather cover of chickens.

REFERENCES

Aerni, V., El Lethey, H. and Wechsler, B. (2000) Effect of foraging material and food form on feather pecking in laying hens. *British Poultry Science* 41, 16–21.

Al Bustany, Z. and Elwinger, K. (1986) Effect of dietary protein concentration on performance of hens selected on low protein diet and grouped according to their early production. *Acta Agriculturae Scandinavica* 36, 264–274.

Al Bustany, Z. and Elwinger, K. (1987a) Response of laying hens to different dietary lysine intakes. A comparison of some commercial hybrids with strains selected on a low protein diet. *Acta Agriculturae Scandinavica* 37, 27–40.

Al Bustany, Z. and Elwinger, K. (1987b) Comparison between barley/fish meal- and maize/soybean meal-based diets with various lysine and protein levels fed to different strains of laying hens. *Acta Agriculturae Scandinavica* 37, 41–49.

Ambrosen, T. and Petersen, V.E. (1997) The influence of protein level in the diet on cannibalism and quality of plumage of layers. *Poultry Science* 76, 559–563.

Anderson, J.O. and Warnick, R.E. (1967) Gross abnormalities in chicks fed amino acid deficient diets. *Poultry Science* 46, 856–862.

Arrazola, A., Mosco, E., Widowski, T., Guerin, M. and Torrey, S. (2017) Does feed restriction lead to fault bar development in broiler breeders? In: Wickens, S., Hubrecht, R. and Golledge, H. (eds) *Measuring Animal Welfare and Applying Scientific Advances – why is sit still so difficult?* UFAW International Animal Welfare Science Symposium, Royal Holloway, University of London, 27–29 June 2017. Universities Federation for Animal Welfare, Wheathampstead, UK.

Aviagen (2013) *Parent Stock Management Manual: Ross 308*. Aviagen Ltd, Huntsville, Alabama.

Baker, D.H. and Molitoris, B.A. (1975) Lack of response to supplemental tin, vanadium, chromium and nickel when added to a purified crystalline amino acid diet for chicks. *Poultry Science* 54, 925–927.

Bilcik, B. and Keeling, L.J. (1999) Changes in feather condition in relation to feather pecking and aggressive behaviour in laying hens. *British Poultry Science* 40, 444–451.

Champe, K.A. and Maurice, D.V. (1984) Plasma sulphur AA in the domestic hen following molt induced by low sodium diet. *Nutrition Reports International* 30, 965.

Daghir, N.J. and Balloun S.L. (1963) Evaluation of the effects of breed on vitamin B6 requirements of chicks. *Journal of Nutrition* 79, 279–288.

De Jong, I.C., Wolthuis-Fillerup, M. and van Emous, R.A. (2009) Development of sexual behaviour in commercially-housed broiler breeders after mixing. *British Poultry Science* 50, 151–160.

Deschutter, A. and Leeson, S. (1986) Feather growth and development. *World's Poultry Science Journal* 42, 259–267.

Edens, F.W., Parkhurst C.R. and Havenstein, G.B. (2001) Housing and selenium influences on feathering in broilers. *Journal of Applied Poultry Research* 10, 128–134.

El Lethey, H., Aerni, V., Jungi, T.W. and Wechsler, B. (2000) Stress and feather pecking in laying hens in relation to housing conditions. *British Poultry Science* 41, 22–28.

Elwinger, K. (1981) Different energy levels and restricted feeding to three strains of SCWL hybrids. 1. Effects on egg production. *Swedish Journal of Agricultural Research* 11, 149–157.

Elwinger, K., Tauson, R. Tufvesson M. and Hartmann, C. (2002) Feeding of layers kept in an organic feed environment. In: WPSA (ed.) *Proceedings 11th European Poultry Conference, Bremen*. Pharma Service, Hannover, Germany, pp. 1–12

Farran, M.T. and Thomas, O.P. (1992) Valine deficiency 1. The effect of feeding a valine deficient diet during the starter period on performance and feather structure of male broiler chicks. *Poultry Science* 71, 1879–1884.

Fisher, M.L., Leeson, S., Morrison, W.D. and Summers, J.D. (1981) Feather growth and feather composition of broiler chickens. *Canadian Journal of Animal Science* 61, 769–773.

Glatz, P.C. (2001) Effect of poor feather cover on feed intake and production of aged laying hens. *Asian–Australasian Journal of Animal Science* 14(4), 553–558.

Hancock, C.E., Bradford, G.D., Emmans, G.C. and Gous, R.M. (1995) The evaluation of the growth parameters of six strains of commercial broiler chickens. *British Poultry Science* 36, 247–264.

Harrap, B.S. and Woods. E.F. (1964) Soluble derivatives of feather keratin. *Biochemical Journal* 49, 8–26.

Hoffmeyer, I. (1969) Feather pecking in pheasants – an ethological approach to the problem. *Danish Review of Game Biology* 6, 1–36.

Jovani, R. and Blas, J. (2004) Adaptive allocation of stress-induced deformities on bird feathers. *Journal of Evolutionary Biology* 17, 294–301.

Jovani, R. and Rohwer, S. (2017) Fault bars in bird feathers: mechanisms, and ecological and evolutionary causes and consequences. *Biological Reviews* 92, 1113–1127.

Kalinowski, A., Moran, E.T. and Wyatt, C. (2003) Methionine and cystine requirements of slow- and fast-feathering male broilers from zero to three weeks of age. *Poultry Science* 82, 1423–1427.

Kemp, D.J. and Rogers, G.E. (1972) Differentiation of avian keratinocytes. Characterization and relationships of the keratin proteins of adult and embryonic feathers and scales. *Biochemistry* 11, 969–975.

King, J.R. and Murphy, M.E. (1984) Fault bars in the feathers of white-crowned sparrows: dietary deficiency or stress of captivity and handling? *The Auk* 101, 168–169.

Kjaer, J.B. and Sørensen, P. (2002) Feather pecking and cannibalism in free-range laying hens as affected by genotype, dietary level of methionine+cystine, light intensity during rearing and age at first access to the range area. *Applied Animal Behaviour Science* 76, 21–39.

Köhler, B., Föhlsch, J., Strube, J. and Lange, K. (2001) Influences of green forage and lighting conditions on egg quality and hen welfare. In: Oester, H. and Wyss, C. (eds) *Proceedings of the 6th European Symposium on Poultry Welfare*. Swiss Branch of the World's Poultry Science Association (WPSA), Zollikofen, Switzerland, pp. 20–21.

LaBrash, L.F. and Scheideler, S.E. (2005) Farm feather condition score survey of commercial laying hens. *Journal of Applied Poultry Research* 14, 740–744.

Leeson, S. and Summers, J.D. (1997) Feeding programs for broilers. In: Leeson, S. and Summers, J.D. (eds) *Commercial Poultry Nutrition*, 2nd edn. University Books, Guelph, Ontario, pp. 207–254.

Leeson, S. and Walsh, T. (2004a) Feathering in commercial poultry. I. Feather growth and composition. *World's Poultry Science Journal* 60, 42–51.

Leeson, S. and Walsh, T. (2004b) Feathering in commercial poultry. II. Factors influencing feather growth and feather loss. *World's Poultry Science Journal* 60, 52–63.

Merat, P. and Coquerelle, G. (1991) The effects of slightly higher or lower than normal incubation temperatures on embryo mortality, post-hatching performance and feathering. *Annales de Zootechnie* 40, 67–72.

Moran, E.T. (1981) Cystine requirements of feather-sexed broiler chickens with sex and age. *Poultry Science* 60, 1056–1061.

Moran, E.T. (1984) Feathers and L-methionine substitutes. *Feed Management* January, 46.

Newton, I. (2010) *The Sparrowhawk*. Poyser, London.

Ostmann, O.W., Ringer, R.K. and Tetzlaff, M. (1963) The anatomy of the feather follicle and its immediate surroundings. *Poultry Science* 42, 957–969.

Peguri, A. and Coon, C. (1993) Effect of feather coverage and temperature on layer performance. *Poultry Science* 72, 1318–1329.

Penz, A.M., Kratzer, F.H. and Rogers, Q.R. (1984) Effect of excess leucine on feather structure and feather composition in the chick. *Nutrition Reports International* 29, 991–995.

Robel, E.J. (1977) A feather abnormality in chicks fed diets deficient in certain amino acids. *Poultry Science* 56, 1968–1971.

Sanders, B.G., Brown, B.G. and Couch, J.R. (1950) A feathering syndrome in chicks after feeding optimal levels of lysine in the absence of arginine. *Proceedings of the Society for Experimental Biology and Medicine* 74, 114–117.

Savory, C.J. (1980) Meal occurrence in Japanese quail in relation to particle size and nutrient density. *Animal Behaviour* 28, 160–171.

Savory, C.J. (1998) Feather pecking damage in growing bantams is influenced by dietary tryptophan concentration but not dietary protein source. *British Poultry Science* 39 (Suppl. 001), 17–18.

Savory, C.J., Mann, J.S. and Macleod, M.G. (1999) Incidence of pecking damage in growing bantams in relation to food form, group size, stocking density, dietary tryptophan concentration and dietary protein source. *British Poultry Science* 40, 579–584.

Schaible, P.J., Davidson, J.A. and Bandemer, S.L. (1947) Cannibalism and feather pecking in chicks as influenced by certain changes in a specific ration. *Poultry Science* 26, 651–656.

Scott, M.L., Holm, E.R. and Reynolds, R.E. (1959) Studies on niacin, riboflavin, choline, manganese and zinc requirements of young ring-necked pheasants for growth, feathering and prevention of leg disorders. *Poultry Science* 38, 1344–1350.

Sirén, M.J. (1963) Cannibalism in cockerels and pheasants. *Acta Veterinaria Scandinavica* 4 (Suppl. 1), 1–47.

Steenfeldt, S., Engberg, R.M. and Kjaer, J.B. (2001) Feeding roughage to laying hens affects egg production, gastro-intestinal parameters and mortality. In: *Proceedings of the 13th European Symposium on Poultry Nutrition*, World's Poultry Science Association, Geel, Belgium, pp. 238–239.

Steenfeldt, S., Kjaer, J. and Engberg, R.M. (2007) Effect of feeding silages or carrots as supplements to laying hens on production performance, nutrient digestibility, gut structure, gut microflora and feather pecking behaviour. *British Poultry Science* 48, 454–468.

Stilborn, H.L., Moran, E.T., Gous, R.M. and Harrison, M.D. (1997) Effect of age on feather amino acid content in two broiler strain crosses and sexes. *Journal of Applied Poultry Research* 6, 205–209.

Stilborn, H.L., Moran, E.T., Gous, R.M. and Harrison, M.D. (2010) Influence of age on carcass (feather-free) amino acid content for two broiler strain-crosses and sexes. *Journal of Applied Poultry Research* 19, 13–23.

Strochlic, D. and Romero, L.M. (2008) The effects of chronic psychological and physical stress on feather replacement in European starlings (*Sturnus vulgaris*). *Comparative Biochemistry and Physiology – Part A: Molecular & Integrative Physiology* 149, 68–79.

Summers, J.D., Leeson, S. and Ferguson, A.E. (1978) Performance and leg condition of caged and floor reared broilers fed diets deficient in selected vitamins and minerals. *Poultry Science* 57, 506–512.

Sunde, M.L. (1972) Zinc requirement for normal feathering of commercial Leghorn-type pullets. *Poultry Science* 51, 1316–1322.

Supplee, W.C. (1966) Feather abnormality in poults fed diet deficient in vitamin E and selenium. *Poultry Science* 45, 852–854.

Supplee, W.C., Combs, G.F. and Blamberg, D.L. (1958) Zinc and potassium effects on bone formation, feathering and growth of pullets. *Poultry Science* 37, 63–67.

Taylor, T.G. (1967) A characteristic feather abnormality in chicks. *Poultry Science* 36, 315.

Tsiagbe, V.K., Kraus, R.J., Benevenga, N.J., Harper, A.E. and Sunde, M.L. (1987) Identification of volatile sulfur derivatives released from feathers of chicks fed diets with various levels of sulfur containing amino acids. *Journal of Nutrition* 117, 1859–1865.

Twining, P.V., Thomas, O.P. and Bossard, E.H. (1976) Number of feathers on litter – another criterion for evaluating adequacy of broiler diets. *Poultry Science* 55, 200–1207.

Urdaneta-Rincon, M. and Leeson, S. (2004) Effect of dietary crude protein and lysine on feather growth in chicks to twenty-one days of age. *Poultry Science* 83, 1713–1717.

Van der Lee, A.G., Hemke, G. and Kwakkel, R.P. (2001) Low density diets improve plumage condition in non-debeaked layers. In: *Proceedings of 13th European Symposium on Poultry Nutrition*, World's Poultry Science Association, Geel, Belgium, pp. 244–245.

Van Emous, R.A. (2015) Body composition and reproduction in broiler breeders: impact of feeding strategies. PhD Thesis, Wageningen University, Wageningen, The Netherlands.

Van Emous, R.A., Kwakkel, R.P., van Krimpen, M.M. and Hendriks, W.H. (2014) Effects of growth patterns and dietary protein levels during rearing on feed intake, eating time, eating rate, behavior, plasma corticosterone concentration, and feather cover in broiler breeder females during the rearing and laying period. *Applied Animal Behaviour Science* 150, 44–54.

Van Emous, R.A., Kwakkel, R.P., van Krimpen, M.M. and Hendriks, W.H. (2015) Effects of dietary protein levels during rearing and dietary energy levels during lay on behaviour and feather cover in broiler breeder females. *Applied Animal Behaviour Science* 168, 45–55.

Van Hierden, Y.M., Korte, S.M., Ruesink, E.W., van Reenen, C.G., Engel, B. *et al.* (2002) Adrenocortical reactivity and central serotonin and dopamine turnover in young chicks from a high and low feather pecking line of laying hens. *Physiology and Behavior* 75, 653–659.

Van Hierden, Y.M., Koolhaas, J.M., de Boer, S.F. and Korte, S.M. (2004) The control of feather pecking by serotonin. *Behavioral Neuroscience* 118, 575–583.

Van Krimpen, M.M. (2008) Impact of nutritional factors on eating behavior and feather damage of laying hens. PhD Thesis, Wageningen University, Wageningen, The Netherlands.

Van Krimpen, M.M., Kwakkel, R.P., Reuvekamp, B.F.J., van der Peet-Schwering, C.M.C., den Hartog, L.A. and Verstegen, M.W.A. (2005) Impact of feeding management on feather pecking in laying hens. *World's Poultry Science Journal* 61, 663–685.

Walser, P. and Pfirter, H.P. (2001) Feed structure influences behaviour of laying hens. In: *Proceedings of the 6th European Symposium on Poultry Welfare*. Swiss Branch of the World's Poultry Science Association (WPSA), Zollikofen, Switzerland, pp. 181–185.

Wheeler, K.B. and Latshaw, J.D. (1981) Sulfur amino-acid requirements and interactions in broilers during two growth periods. *Poultry Science* 60, 228–236.

Wyatt, R.D., Hamilton, P.B. and Burmeister, H.R. (1975) Altered feathering of chicks caused by T-2 toxin. *Poultry Science* 54, 1042–1045.

Wylie, L.M., Robertson, G.W. and Hocking, P.M. (2003) Effects of dietary protein concentration and specific amino acids on body weight, body composition and feather growth in young turkeys. *British Poultry Science* 44, 75–87.

CHAPTER 12
Strengthening the Inside: Effect of Nutrition on Gut Health and Maintenance and Its Impact on the Integument Integrity

Sunday A. Adedokun* and Opeyemi C. Olojede

University of Kentucky, Lexington, Kentucky, USA

ABSTRACT

The gastrointestinal tract (GIT) of poultry is equipped to perform several important functions. One of these functions is the protection of the underlying structures of the entire digestive tract and minimization of the translocation of materials that may be inimical to the health of the bird. The GIT also plays an important role in the digestion and absorption of nutrients and houses a vast array of microbiota with the potential to impact gut health. Strengthening the GIT involves early and proper establishment of the gut's physical, microbiological, secretory and immunological components to build strong intestinal barriers against potentially harmful organisms. As such, a strong and healthy gut, characterized by proper intestinal functionality, integrity and immunity, is essential for superior performance and overall well-being of the bird. To meet this goal, timely and balanced nutrition is important and is essential early in the life of the birds.

The objective of this chapter is to discuss the impact of nutrition on the health of the GIT of poultry. Nutrition approaches for fostering a healthy gut include the maintenance of a healthy mucous layer throughout the GIT. Research has shown that adequate supply of dietary protein (amino acid) and specific carbohydrates are important for a healthy mucous layer. Also, early nutrition, both *in ovo* feeding and access to feed within the first 24 h post-hatch, has been shown to quicken the development and the establishment of the GIT and its associated organs. A healthy inside is a reflection of the integrity and functionality of the tight junction proteins that selectively allow the passage of nutrients across the intestinal epithelium layer into the mucosal layer while excluding agents that may be harmful to the bird. Research continues to show that

*tayo.adedokun@uky.edu

cultivating a healthy microbial population in the GIT is important for the bird to thrive. Feed supplements such as pre- and probiotics have been supplemented to poultry diets for this purpose. However, the total withdrawal of antibiotics from poultry feed creates new challenges as well as more opportunities for cutting-edge research on the best approaches for improving gut health without the use of antibiotics.

INTRODUCTION

A healthy gut is a healthy bird. Today's birds have been developed to perform at an incredibly high level for the purpose for which they were bred and selected (broiler, turkey and ducks for meat and laying hens for eggs). Because of this, birds that are selected for rapid growth rate and high feed efficiency have high feed consumption levels. For example, a day-old broiler chick is expected to weigh 2.7–3.1 kg by day 42 with feed consumption of 4.5–5.1 kg. Also, an average modern turkey is expected to attain body weight of 21.8–25.2 kg by week 22 with feed intake of 58.5–66.1 kg, depending on the breed. This shows that the quantity of feed that passes through the entire gastrointestinal tract (GIT) of these birds is incredibly high. In addition to this, feeds that are given to poultry consist of several ingredients from different sources with different physico-chemical properties. Aside from being sources of nutrients to the birds, feed and water (as well as materials from the environment, e.g. litter) may be sources of some anti-nutritional factors or carriers of microbes such as fungi (mycotoxins) with potentials to be pathogenic. The GIT, like any other tract, is open to the outside and, if not adequately protected, any interaction with pathogenic microbes has the potential to result in the translocation of these pathogens into the blood.

The GIT of birds has been reported to undergo active morphological, cellular and molecular development towards the end of the incubation period with a relatively higher rate of increase in intestinal weight compared with the weight of the developing embryo (Uni, 2006). This process of intestinal growth and development continues post-hatch. Furthermore, the establishment of microbiota in the intestine progresses quite rapidly within the first few days until the microbiota population stabilizes. All of these indicate that the quality of the diet and water, as well as the environment where the birds are raised, in the first few days could impact the long-term health of the GIT.

The use of phytase, carbohydrase, or protease (or a combination of these) has the potential to reduce digesta viscosity and increase digestion and absorption of nutrients (Adeola and Cowieson, 2011), thereby resulting in a reduction in the level of nutrients that are available to support the growth and proliferation of pathogenic organisms post the midgut (Bedford, 2000). Strengthening the GIT of birds requires concerted interdisciplinary research efforts from nutritionists, geneticists, pathologists and immunologists. With an increasing array of feed additives and supplements that are commercially available today, there is a need for further screening and research to identify the active compound, its mode of action, dosage level, combination(s) and appropriate timing for their use in poultry.

GASTROINTESTINAL TRACT

The GIT is an open-ended, epithelium-lined tube that runs from the beak to the cloaca. One of the primary functions of the GIT is to digest food into its basic components for absorption and utilization by the bird. From the beak to the cloaca, the GIT is lined with a mucous membrane, which allows it to interact continuously with dietary antigens and diverse microorganisms (DeSesso and Jacobson, 2001). According to Turner (2009), complex multicellular organisms interface with their external environments at multiple sites, via the mucosa. The airways, oral cavity, digestive tract, genitourinary tract and the skin are lined by mucous membrane, but the GIT is said to have the largest mucosal surface. The GIT is composed of four concentric layers, with the intestinal mucosa being the innermost layer. Within the mucosa is a single layer of columnar epithelial cells, as well as the underlying lamina propria and muscular mucosae (Turner, 2009). The intestinal epithelial cells cover the mucosa and form cellular barriers that separate the internal from the external environment. This requires that they develop distinct cell surface domains (mainly enterocytes, goblet cells, Paneth cells, endocrine cells, caveolated and cup cells, M cells, stem cells and intraepithelial lymphocytes), which fosters an interaction through adhesive complexes between the cells (Santos and Perdue, 2000; Matter and Balda, 2007). The epithelial cells serve several functions in the intestinal tract. The junctional complexes act as a selectively permeable barrier, allowing for the absorption of nutrients, electrolytes and water from the intestinal lumen into circulation (blood), and prevent the passage of noxious toxins, antigens and intestinal flora into the blood.

The concept of permeability can be attributed to the structure of the membrane (composition, charge, thickness, integrity) that enables the passage of a solute by unmediated diffusion. Intestinal epithelium mediates its selective permeability by a series of intercellular junctions and fluid (as well as solute) movement either through transcellular or paracellular pathways (Laukoetter *et al.*, 2006; Groschwitz and Hogan, 2009). Transcellular permeability is generally associated with the transport of energy-dependent macromolecules from the luminal space to the interstitial space and is predominantly regulated by active transporters for amino acids (AA), electrolytes, short-chain fatty acids and sugars (Groschwitz and Hogan, 2009; Goddard and Iruela-Arispe, 2013). Paracellular permeability, on the other hand, maintains barrier function by allowing transport in the space between epithelial cells. This action is maintained through the formation of complex protein–protein networks (Groschwitz and Hogan, 2009) that are bound together by junctional complexes located at the most apical part of the lateral membrane: the tight junction (TJ), the adherens junctions (AJ) and the desmosomes (Tsukita *et al.*, 2001). These complexes consist of actin-binding proteins that interact with adjacent cells and intracellularly with adaptor proteins that link to the actin cytoskeleton through cytoplasmic scaffolding proteins. They mediate adhesion and provide mechanical strength, restrict diffusion across epithelia and regulate signalling pathways that control cell proliferation, polarization and differentiation (Matter and Balda, 2007; Groschwitz and Hogan, 2009). In conjunction with the epithelial cells mediating an efficient intestinal integrity of the GIT is the presence of a diverse and complex but dynamic community of microorganisms that confers protection against potential pathogens via a mucosal immune system (Bauer *et al.*, 2006). Each region of the GIT develops its own unique microbial profile, and this community becomes more complex with age.

Adherens junctions (AJs), along with desmosomes, are protein complexes on the lateral membrane that form distinct complexes that are linked to the intermediate filament cytoskeleton. AJs are composed of cadherin–caterin interactions. The epithelial cadherins (E-cadherins) promote a cell–cell adhesion by forming homotypical interactions with cadherins of neighbouring cells (Groschwitz and Hogan, 2009; Turner, 2009). They also interact directly with catenins, by linking the AJ to the cytoskeletal network through actin-binding proteins or other adaptor proteins such as afadin. Through these cadherin–catenin complexes, AJs form a mechanical linkage of adjacent cells, maintain cell polarity and regulate epithelial migration and proliferation. However, loss of AJs results in the disruption of cell–cell matrix with perturbed intestinal epithelial proliferation and migration (Matter and Balda, 2003; Groschwitz and Hogan, 2009; Goddard and Iruela-Arispe, 2013). Furthermore, AJs are required for the assembly of the tight junctions (TJs), which seal the paracellular space and provide the epithelial tissue diffusion barrier that is critical for the normal functioning of organs and tissues. Groschwitz and Hogan (2009) referred to TJs as adhesive junctional complexes in mammalian epithelial cells composed of dynamic multicellular complexes that function as a selective barrier, which limits solutes flux through the intercellular space while preventing the translocation of luminal antigens, microorganisms and their toxins. Therefore, it is often described as the rate-limiting step in trans-epithelial transport and mucosal permeability (Turner, 2009). These barriers are maintained by the membrane proteins, which can be grouped into two classes: single domain transmembrane proteins (JAMs, Crb-3) and four domain transmembrane proteins (occludin, tricellulin and claudins) (Matter and Balda, 2003). It is interesting to note the complexities involved in the development of the GIT in order to efficiently perform the function of nutrient and energy absorption while preventing the translocation of materials that may be inimical to the health of the animal. Despite this, these defensive mechanisms could be compromised under a high level of insult (physical, chemical, or biological damage) leading to a weaker defence system in the GIT. This could lead to a decrease in growth and performance (productivity), morbidity, or death, depending on the severity of the challenge.

STRESS

Maintaining a uniquely balanced microflora population is essential for the health and well-being of the GIT (Laukoetter *et al.*, 2006). During periods of normal health, resident microbiomes in the GIT of chickens play an important role in growth and development through the production of energy-rich short-chain fatty acids, the development of the villus and crypt morphology, nutrient utilization and absorption and the deconstruction of dietary polysaccharides (Muramatsu *et al.*, 1994; Bedford, 2000; Yeoman *et al.*, 2012). The effect of these, under normal conditions, strengthens the integrity of the GIT and subsequently the viability of the host. Similarly, proper functioning of the GIT is dependent on the intestinal mucosa, which is lined by a monolayer of epithelial cells that come into contact with the external environment and becomes a barrier protecting the body against harmful factors (Sikora and Grzesiuk, 2007). Thus, this balanced state of intestinal secretion and permeability, actively maintained by neural and immune factors, helps to ensure that the lumen of the gut lining maintains the commensal bacteria. The influence of stress on mucosal barrier function in the GIT is increasingly being recognized. Under physiological circumstances, the intestinal mucosa sets a barrier between internal and external environments and prevents excessive penetration of antigens through the epithelial layer that might result in inappropriate immune stimulations. It could be expected that stressors on the digestive system, or in an event of defective protective response, might influence the normal flora colonizing the GIT, resulting in a breach in the intestinal barrier, hence a potential negative consequence. Several studies, using intestinal perfusion techniques, have revealed that severe physical and/or biological stress can cause gastrointestinal dysfunction, bacterial translocation and an increase in intestinal permeability (Santos and Perdue, 2000; Söderholm and Perdue, 2001). In animal models, acute stress has been shown to induce enhanced intestinal epithelial permeability to macromolecules (Söderholm *et al.*, 2002), increase fluid and electrolyte transport (Saunders *et al.*, 1994; Santos and Perdue, 2000), disrupt indigenous microflora (Bailey and Coe, 1999; Burkholder *et al.*, 2008) and decrease the overall integrity of intestinal epithelium (Söderholm *et al.*, 2002; Burkholder *et al.*, 2008).

Anything that causes stress endangers life, therefore the ability of the animal to adapt and resist such stress or stressor(s) is an important prerequisite for life and survival (Selye, 1950). A classic knowledge is that stress initiates a very complex set of responses with many interacting factors determining the outcome. In particular, once the epithelial surface has been compromised, through either direct destruction or invasion of bacteria, the mucosal immune system that is capable of responding selectively or specifically against a myriad of threats associated with the GIT is activated. In response to this, effector cells of immune reactions (lymphocytes, eosinophils, mast cells, neutrophils, macrophages and dendritic cells) are activated secreting a wide array of mediators that influence intestinal physiology either through enterocytes or activation of the enteric nervous system (Santos and Perdue, 1998). A large body of evidence suggests that intestinal barrier dysfunction is associated with several diseases, which are usually due to epithelial defects, such as incomplete polarization, brush border and actin cytoskeleton disruption, accelerated crypt–villus migration and eventually apoptosis (Jankowski *et al.*, 1994; Podolsky, 1999; Groschwitz and Hogan, 2009; Turner, 2009). Furthermore, the disruption in the intestinal barrier is usually followed by an increase in the numbers of pro-inflammatory cytokines, such as tumour necrotic factor (TNF) and interferon gamma (IFN-γ) and interleukin-10 (IL-10) as well as immunoregulatory responses.

Similarly to cells, tissues and physiological fluids in the body of an animal exposed to any form of stress (arising from an insult or challenge) at the intestinal level will result in the disruption of the balance between the production and elimination of the reactive oxygen species (ROS) (Georgieva *et al.*, 2011). The high level of ROS in the intestinal cells sets into motion the destruction of the polyunsaturated fatty acids in the membrane of cells, leading to peroxidation, with eventual production of several products with malondialdehyde (MDA) being one of the prominent end products of this reaction. Once this process continues, the integrity of the cell membrane is compromised, and could result in nutrient malabsorption, morbidity, or mortality. In addition to physical, biological (e.g. *Eimeria* sp. or *Clostridium perfringens* challenge), or chemical (e.g. dexamethasone challenge) stressors, it has been shown that dietary deficiencies in certain nutrients can increase the susceptibility of poultry to oxidative stress (Bun *et al.*, 2011; Georgieva *et al.*, 2011; Gao *et al.*, 2017). Loss of intestinal integrity and functionality will lead to malabsorption, a decrease in performance, bacterial translocation, product (meat and egg) contamination, morbidity and, in some cases, the death of the bird.

NUTRITION

The use of antibiotics in farm animals has been under a lot of scrutiny. Recent studies have attributed the current epidemic of bacterial resistance to its overuse, and suggest that it poses certain hazards to human and animal health. However, for a long time, antibiotics were referred to as growth promoters in the livestock production. This dates back to the 1940s when peer-reviewed articles reported the growth-promoting effect of administering antibiotics to chicks (Moore *et al.*, 1946; Stokstad *et al.*, 1949), which they discovered in an attempt to find an inexpensive substitute source of vitamin B_{12} as a dietary supplement for poultry. The administration of these antibiotics became a routine procedure in the commercial setting for its effectiveness in promoting growth and feed efficiency at low levels but also to control epidemics of diseases in large groups of animals (Gustafson and Bowen, 1997; McEwen, 2006). Meanwhile, the profound commercial success of rearing food animals in large numbers in a confined space to meet the needs of billions of people poses a threat in terms of what is required for the optimum health of these rapidly growing birds. Under such conditions, transmission of infectious agents and other environmental stressors increases; thus the need to use antibiotics prophylactically to protect these animals by controlling the diseases, rather than after the disease is evident (Gustafson and Bowen, 1997). To compensate for the restriction on antibiotics use, several measures have been adopted in the prevention and control of many infectious diseases. Special emphasis is placed on finding alternatives for improving bird health, by modulating the immune system of chickens through several practices, including vaccination programmes, breeding, husbandry practices and nutrition (Khan *et al.*, 2012).

There is much evidence linking diet and the maintenance of the intestinal mucosa integrity. Recent advances have uncovered some of the mechanisms by which physiological and immunological stimuli affect components of the intestinal barrier. Studies have shown that the strongest determinant of the gut microbial profile is the host's diet (Pan and Yu, 2014; Munyaka *et al.*, 2016; Dong *et al.*, 2017). Factors such as diet composition, nutrient density, feed physical characteristics, feed processing techniques and feed additives play significant roles in the dynamics of the GIT microflora. One possible approach for an improvement in this area is to elucidate the effects of different nutrient regimens in stressed or diseased birds. Based on available information in the literature, we know that nutrients can modulate immune response through several mechanisms. These include the development of immune cells and tissues necessary for synthesizing effector cells, proliferation of certain pathogens by modifying the population of microorganisms in the GIT, providing substrates for the construction of cells and molecules such as leucocytes that respond to infectious challenges, and indirectly activating the endocrine system (Klasing, 1998). The early days of a chick's life are especially crucial for the development of the gut immune system. The chicks are vulnerable at that time, due to the rapid development and immaturity of the host defence (Uni, 2006). This has led to a movement towards strengthening the gut of a chick to ensure efficient maturation of the GIT post-hatch as well as the development of lymphoid organs by the administration of nutrients into the amnion through *in ovo* feeding (Gao *et al.*, 2017). Lilburn and Loeffler (2015) summarized the advantages of *in ovo* feeding to include an increase in brush-border enzyme activities, intestinal nutrient and glucose absorption, villus surface area, as well as an increase in the expression of some brush-border membrane transporters (Tako *et al.*, 2004, 2005; Smirnov *et al.*, 2006; Foye *et al.*, 2007). This epigenetic effect is said to change the structure of the intestinal epithelium and enhance yolk absorption by the small intestines (Uni, 1998), increases the chances of the bird to resist enteric infection like necrotic enteritis (Beal *et al.*, 2006; Keerqin *et al.*, 2017) and accelerates growth performance (Bakyaraj *et al.*, 2012).

The remarkable advances in immunology and nutrition in recent decades have shed more light on the effect of various nutrients on specific GIT functions, including immune response, and how they influence host resistance to infection. One of the major causes of immunodeficiency globally has been attributed to protein and energy malnutrition (Field *et al.*, 2002; Ruth and Field, 2013). Studies have shown that an adequate nutritional regimen is essential to maintain a healthy gut, and deficiencies in dietary protein (or amino acids, AA), which reduces plasma concentration of AA, can suppress immune response by decreasing lymphocyte number, overall leucocyte count and splenic cell proliferation stimulated with phytohaemagglutinin-M (Payne *et al.*, 1990; Kidd, 2004; Li *et al.*, 2007). Moreover, during immunological stress, immune system activation and inflammation use up the available protein (needed for growth) for the production of cytokines (interleukin-1, interleukin-6 and tumour necrosis factor-α), which alter the overall protein metabolism. As a result, normal metabolic processes are discouraged, but this can be redeemed by optimizing AA levels in the diet. Thus, attention has been directed to the substantial role of individual AA on the integrity, growth and development of the intestinal epithelium and its associated immune function. In particular, the roles of glutamine, arginine, tryptophan and cysteine (Wu *et al.*, 1999; Le Floc'h *et al.*, 2004; Gao *et al.*, 2017) have been investigated. Specifically, Gao *et al.* (2017) showed that *in ovo* feeding of arginine influenced the development of lymphoid organs in broiler chicks, while Tan *et al.* (2014, 2015) showed that L-arginine supplementation could regulate the immune function in challenged birds. Similarly, Lee *et al.* (2002) reported that arginine had a positive influence on chicken cellular response to infectious bronchitis virus and that it activated the mechanistic target of rapamycin (mTOR) pathway in intestinal epithelium cells with the potential to function in the repair of damaged intestinal epithelium (Ban *et al.*, 2004). Glutamine is said to: (i) provide sufficient amounts of ATP used by mesenteric lymph node lymphocytes (Wu *et al.*, 1991; Kim *et al.*, 2007), essential for the proliferation and function of lymphocytes (Field *et al.*, 2002); (ii) enhance phagocytic activity of macrophages and the production of cytokines and antibodies by T and B lymphocytes, respectively (Parry-Billings *et al.*, 1990; Kim *et al.*, 2007); (iii) enhance the digestion and absorption of macromolecules by activating the signalling pathway in the GIT via the gut–brain axis (Wu *et al.*, 2014); and (iv) improve chick growth performance (Bartell and Batal, 2007). Threonine is another important AA that is abundant in the mucin that lines the entire GIT. An adequate dietary level of threonine has been shown to enhance intestinal integrity in poultry (Dong *et al.*, 2017).

It has been documented that certain minerals enhance intestinal health. Adequate levels of zinc supplementation in poultry diet have been reported to reduce the formation and the impact of oxidative damage in the intestine of broilers challenged with *Eimeria* species (Bun *et al.*, 2011; Georgieva *et al.*, 2011). In the same line, several studies have confirmed the effect of adequate dietary levels of selenium, nucleotides and long-chain polyunsaturated fatty acids, as well as vitamins A, C, and E in modulating the host defence against infectious pathogens (Field *et al.*, 2002). This demonstrates the need for nutrient-directed management practices of immune-mediated diseases (Field *et al.*, 2002). Furthermore, inasmuch as it is impossible to raise chickens in a perfect environment that is completely devoid of pathogenic organisms, it is essential to minimize their negative effects on poultry GITs via nutritional means. In order to maximize digestion and absorption of nutrients from the diets given to poultry, efforts should also be made to reduce the amount of nutrients that escape hydrolytic digestion in the midgut. The presence of a large quantity of undigested and unabsorbed nutrients and energy in the hindgut is inimical to the health of the GIT of the bird. Feeding of highly digestible diets is one of the ways in which this could be achieved (Bedford, 2000; Moran, 2014). Highly digestible diets allow for most of the nutrients in the diets to be digested and absorbed prior to reaching the hindgut, where most of the pathogenic microbes are found. In addition to this, more than 70% of feeds given to poultry are plant-based; the use of exogenous enzymes such as phytase (phytate and phytic acid breakdown for improved P digestibility), protease (protein digestion) and carbohydrases (non-starch polysaccharide, NSP, breakdown) is essential (Adeola and Cowieson, 2011).One of the ways through which the NSP-degrading enzymes function is by reducing digesta viscosity, which subsequently allows endogenous enzymes to gain better access to the digesta and hence increases nutrient and energy digestibility. Secondly, the passage rate of the digesta is slowed down, allowing for sufficient time for digestion and absorption to take place. The combination of these actions will lead to a reduction in the quantity and quality of nutrient and energy that reach the hindgut, thereby denying pathogenic organisms the needed nutritional support (Bedford, 2000; Moran, 2014). Furthermore, the action of this enzyme could result in a reduction in the level of moisture in the excreta and subsequently in the litter. This has the tendency to reduce the build-up of pathogenic organisms in the litter.

SUMMARY

Understanding the effects of stress on metabolism and nutrient digestibility, as well as effective stress induction models, is essential to any researcher interested in further delineating the effects of nutrients on the integrity of the GIT of poultry. Research has clearly established that partitioning of nutrients away from growth towards host defence becomes a priority during an infection or stress-related events. Thus, novel strategies to minimize the impact of these stressors on poultry GIT health through adequate levels of dietary nutrients and necessary dietary supplements in poultry diets combined with effective management strategies will be the key to maintaining a healthy gut. Furthermore, emphasis should be placed on the nature, contents, as well as nutrient densities of the feed that is given to the birds. These have the potential to influence the density and diversity of the microbiota in the GIT as well as the immuno-modulatory effects of these nutrients on the immunity and overall health of the chicken. Applications of these strategies can strengthen the health of the GIT, increase feed efficiencies, and improve food safety.

REFERENCES

Adeola, O. and Cowieson, A.J. (2011) Opportunities and challenges in using exogenous enzymes to improve nonruminant animal production. Board-invited Review. *Journal of Animal Science* 89(10), 3189–3218.

Bailey, M.T. and Coe, C.L. (1999) Maternal separation disrupts the integrity of the intestinal microflora in infant rhesus monkeys. *Developmental Psychobiology* 35,146–155.

Bakyaraj, S., Bhanja, S.K., Majumdar, S. and Dash, B. (2012) Modulation of post-hatch growth and immunity through *in ovo* supplemented nutrients in broiler chickens. *Journal of the Science of Food and Agriculture* 92, 313–320.

Ban, H., Shigemitsu, K., Yamatsuji, T., Haisa, M., Nakajo, T. *et al.* (2004) Arginine and leucine regulate p70 S6 kinase and 4E-BP1 in intestinal epithelial cells. *International Journal of Molecular Medicine* 13, 537–543.

Bao, X., Feng, Z., Yao, J., Li, T. and Yin, Y. (2017) Role of dietary amino acids and their metabolites in pathogenesis of inflammatory bowel disease. *Mediators of Inflammation* 2017, 1–9.

Bartell, S.M. and Batal, A.B. (2007) The effect of supplemental glutamine on growth performance, development of the gastrointestinal tract, and humoral immune response of broilers. *Poultry Science* 86, 1940–1947.

Bauer, E., Williams, B.A., Smidt, H. Verstegen, M.W. and Mosenthin, R. (2006) Influence of the gastrointestinal microbiota on development of the immune system in young animals. *Current Issues in Intestinal Microbiology* 7, 35–52.

Beal, R.K., Powers, C., Davison, T.F., Barrow, P.A. and Smith, A.L. (2006) Clearance of enteric *Salmonella enterica* serovar *Typhimurium* in chickens is independent of B-cell function. *Infectious Immunology* 74, 1442–1444.

Bedford, M.R. (2000) Removal of antibiotic growth promoters from poultry diets: implications and strategies to minimise subsequent problems. *World's Poultry Science* 56, 347–365.

Bun, S.D., Guo, Y.M., Guo, F.C., Ji, F. and Cao, H. (2011) Influence of organic zinc supplementation on the antioxidant status and immune responses of broilers challenged with *Eimeria tenella*. *Poultry Science* 90, 1220–1226.

Burkholder, K.M., Thompson, K.L., Einstein, M.E., Applegate, T.J. and Patterson, J.A. (2008) Influence of stressors on normal intestinal microbiota, intestinal morphology, and susceptibility to *Salmonella enteritidis* colonization in broilers. *Poultry Science* 87, 1734–1741.

DeSesso, J.M. and Jacobson, C.F. (2001) Anatomical and physiological parameters affecting gastrointestinal absorption in humans and rats. *Food and Chemical Toxicology* 39, 209–228.

Dong, X.Y., Azzam, M.M.M. and Zou, X.T. (2017) Effects of dietary threonine supplementation on intestinal barrier function and gut microbiota of laying hens. *Poultry Science* 96, 3654–3663. doi: 10.3382/ps/pex185

Field, C.J., Johnson, I.R. and Schley, P.D. (2002) Nutrients and their role in host resistance to infection. *Journal of Leukocyte Biology* 71, 6–32.

Foye, O.T., Ferket, P.R. and Uni, Z. (2007) The effects of *in ovo* feeding arginine, B-hydroxy-B-methyl-butyrate, and protein on jejunal digestive and absorption activity in embryonic and neonatal turkey poults. *Poultry Science* 86, 2343–2349.

Gao, T., Zhao, M.M., Zhang, L., Li, J.L., Yu, L.L. *et al.* (2017) Effect of *in ovo* feeding of L-arginine on the development of lymphoid organs and small intestinal immune barrier function in posthatch broilers. *Animal Feed Science and Technology* 225, 8–19.

Georgieva, N.V., Gabrashanska, M., Koinarski, V. and Yaneva, Z. (2011) Zinc supplementation against *Eimeria acervulina*-induced oxidative damage in broiler chickens. *Veterinary Medicine International* 2011, 1–7.

Goddard, L.M. and Iruela-Arispe, M.L. (2013) Cellular and molecular regulation of vascular permeability. *Thrombosis and Haemostasis* 109, 407–415.

Groschwitz, K.R. and Hogan, S.P. (2009) Intestinal barrier function: molecular regulation and disease pathogenesis. *Journal of Allergy Clinical Immunology* 124, 3–20.

Gustafson, R.H. and Bowen, R.E. (1997) Antibiotic use in animal agriculture. *Journal of Applied Microbiology* 83, 531–541.

Jankowski, J.A., Goodlad, R.A. and Wright, N.A. (1994) Maintenance of normal intestinal mucosa: function, structure, and adaptation. *Gut* 35, S1–S4.

Keerqin, C., Wu, S.B., Svihus, B., Swick, R., Morgan, N. and Choct, M. (2017) An early feeding regime and a high-density amino acid diet on growth performance of broilers under subclinical necrotic enteritis challenge. *Animal Nutrition* 3, 25–32.

Khan, R.U., Rahman, Z.U., Nikousefat, Z., Javdani, M., Tufarelli, V. *et al.* (2012) Immunomodulating effects of vitamin E in broilers. *World's Poultry Science Journal* 68, 31–40.

Kidd, M.T. (2004) Nutritional modulation of immune function in broilers. *Poultry Science* 83, 650–657.

Kim, S.W., Mateo, R.D., Yin, Y.L. and Wu, G. (2007) Functional amino acids and fatty acids for enhancing production performance of sows and piglets. *Asian–Australasian Journal of Animal Sciences* 20, 295–306.

Klasing, K.C. (1998) Nutritional modulation of resistance to infectious diseases. *Poultry Science* 77, 1119–1125.

Laukoetter, M., Bruewer, G.M. and Nusrat, A. (2006) Regulation of the intestinal epithelial barrier by the apical junctional complex. *Current Opinion in Gastroenterology* 22, 85–89.

Lee, J.E., Austic, R.E., Naqi, S.A., Golemboski, K.A. and Dietert, R.R. (2002) Dietary arginine intake alters avian leukocyte population distribution during infectious bronchitis challenge. *Poultry Science* 81, 793–798.

Le Floc'h, N., Melchior, D. and Obled, C. (2004) Modifications of protein and amino acid metabolism during inflammation and immune system activation. *Livestock Production Science* 87, 37–45.

Li, P., Yin, Y.L., Li, D., Kim, S.W. and Wu. G. (2007) Amino acids and immune function. *British Journal of Nutrition* 98, 237–252.

Lilburn, M.S. and Loeffler, S. (2015) Early intestinal growth and development in poultry. *Poultry Science* 94, 1569–1576.

Matter, K. and Balda, M.S. (2003) Signaling to and from tight junctions. *Nature Reviews Molecular Cell Biology* 4, 225–236.

Matter, K. and Balda, M.S. (2007) Epithelial tight junctions, gene expression and nucleo-junctional interplay. *Journal of Cell Science* 120, 1505–1511.

McEwen, S. (2006) Antibiotic use in animal agriculture: What have we learned and where are we going? *Animal Biotechnology* 17, 239–250.

Moore, P.R., Evenson, A., Luckey, T.D., McCoy, E., Elvehjem, C.A. and Hart, E.B. (1946) Use of sulfasuxidine, streptothricin, and streptomycin in nutritional studies with the chick. *Journal of Biological Chemistry* 165, 437–441.

Moran, E.T. (2014) Intestinal events and nutritional dynamics predisposes *Clostridium perfringes* virulence in broilers. *Poultry Science* 93, 3028–3036.

Munyaka, P.M., Nandha, N.K., Kiarie, E., Nyachoti, C.M. and Khafpour, E. (2016) Impact of combined β-glucanase and xylanase enzymes on growth performance, nutrient utilization and gut microbiota in broiler chickens fed corn or wheat-based diets. *Poultry Science* 95, 528–540.

Muramatsu, T., Nakajima, S. and Okumura, J. (1994) Modification of energy metabolism by the presence of the gut microflora in the chicken. *British Journal of Nutrition* 71, 709–717.

Pan, D. and Yu, Z. (2014) Intestinal microbiome of poultry and its interaction with host and diet. *Gut Microbes* 5, 108–119.

Parry-Billings, M., Calder, P.C., Newsholme, E.A. and Evans, J. (1990) Does glutamine contribute to immunosuppression after major burns? *Lancet* 336, 523–525.

Payne, C.J., Scott, T.R., Dick, J.W. and Glick, B. (1990) Immunity to *Pasteurella multocida* in protein-deficient chickens. *Poultry Science* 69, 2134–2142.

Podolsky, D.K. (1999) Innate mechanisms of mucosal defense and repair: the best offense is a good defense. *American Journal of Physiology – Gastrointestinal and Liver Physiology* 277(3), G495–G499.

Ruth, M.R. and Field, C.J. (2013) The immune modifying effects of amino acids on gut-associated lymphoid tissue. *Journal of Animal Science and Biotechnology* 4, 1–10.

Santos, J. and Perdue, M.H. (1998) Immunological regulation of intestinal epithelial transport. *Digestion* 59, 404–408.

Santos, J. and Perdue, M.H. (2000) Stress and neuroimmune regulation of gut mucosal function. *Gut* 47 (Suppl. 4), iv49–iv51.

Saunders, P.R., Kosecka, U., McKay, D.M. and Perdue, M.H. (1994) Acute stressors stimulate ion secretion and increase epithelial permeability in rat intestine. *American Journal of Physiology* 267, G794–G799.

Selye, H. (1950) Stress and the general adaptation syndrome. *British Medical Journal* 1, 1383–1392.

Sikora, A. and Grzesiuk, E. (2007) Heat shock response in gastrointestinal tract. *Journal of Physiology and Pharmacology* 58, 43–62.

Smirnov, A., Tako, E., Ferket, P.R. and Uni, Z. (2006) Mucin gene expression and mucin content in the chicken intestinal goblet cells are affected by *in ovo* feeding of carbohydrates. *Poultry Science* 85, 669– 673.

Söderholm, J.D. and Perdue, M.H. (2001) II. Stress and intestinal barrier function. *American Journal of Physiology – Gastrointestinal and Liver Physiology* 280, G7–G13.

Söderholm, J.D., Olaison, G., Peterson, K.H., Franzen, L.E., Lindmark, T. *et al.* (2002) Augmented increase in tight junction permeability by luminal stimuli in the non-inflamed ileum of Crohn's disease. *Gut* 50, 307–313.

Stokstad, E.L.R., Jukes, T.H., Pierce, J., Page, A.C. Jr and Franklin, A.L. (1949) The multiple nature of the animal protein factor. *Journal of Biological Chemistry* 180, 647–654.

Tako, E., Ferket, P.R. and Uni, Z. (2004) Effects of *in ovo* feeding of carbohydrates and B-hydroxybutryate–B-methylbutryate on the development of chicken intestine. *Poultry Science* 83, 2023–2028.

Tako, E.P., Ferket, P.R. and Uni, Z. (2005) Changes in chicken intestinal zinc exporter mRNA expression and small intestine functionality following intra-amniotic zinc-methionine administration. *Journal of Nutritional Biochemistry* 16, 339–346.

Tan, J., Liu, S., Guo, Y., Applegate, T.J. and Eicher, S.D. (2014) Dietary L-arginine supplementation attenuates lipopolysaccharide-induced inflammatory response in broiler chickens. *British Journal of Nutrition* 111, 1394–1404.

Tan, J., Guo, Y., Applegate, T.J, Du, E. and Zhao, X. (2015) L-Arginine regulates immune functions in chickens immunized with intermediate strain of infectious bursal disease vaccine. *Japan Poultry Science* 52, 101–108.

Tsukita, S., Furuse, M. and Itoh, M. (2001) Multifunctional strands in tight junctions. *Nature Reviews. Molecular Cell Biology* 2, 285–293.

Turner, J.R. (2009) Intestinal mucosal barrier function in health and disease. *Nature Reviews. Immunology* 9, 799–809.

Uni, Z. (1998) Impact of early nutrition on poultry: review of presentations. *Journal of Applied Poultry Research* 7, 452–455.

Uni, Z. (2006) Early development of small intestinal function. In: Perry, G.C. (ed.) *Avian Gut Function in Health and Disease*. CAB International, Wallingford, UK, pp. 29–42.

Wu, G.Y., Field, C.J. and Marliss, E.B. (1991) Glutamine and glucose metabolism in rat splenocytes and mesenteric lymph node lymphocytes. *American Journal of Physiology – Endocrinology and Metabolism* 260, E141–E147.

Wu, G., Flynn, N.E., Flynn, S.P., Jolly, C.A. and Davis, P.K. (1999) Dietary protein or arginine deficiency impairs constitutive and inducible nitric oxide synthesis by young rats. *Journal of Nutrition* 129, 1347–1354.

Wu, G., Bazer, F.W., Dai, Z., Li, D., Wang, J. and Wu, Z. (2014) Amino acid nutrition in animals: protein synthesis and beyond. *Annual Review of Animal Biosciences* 2, 387–417.

Yeoman, C.J., Chia, N., Jeraldo, P., Sipos, M., Goldenfeld, N.D. and White, B.A. (2012) The microbiome of the chicken gastrointestinal tract. *Animal Health Reserve Review* 13, 89–99.

CHAPTER 13
Management Practices to Prevent Abnormal Feather Loss in Broiler Breeders

Otto A. van Tuijl*
Jannelandseweg 17, 4661 GC Halsteren, The Netherlands

ABSTRACT

This chapter discusses management factors in broiler breeders that can trigger abnormal feathering and unwanted feather damage, such that the birds are unable to maintain good feather cover at all times. Management practices to ensure good feed access include the following.

- Birds have correct feeder and drinker space.
- Feed and water are available immediately the lights come on in the morning.
- Feed distribution time does not exceed 3 min, if necessary filling the system from several locations in order to achieve the correct distribution time.
- Feed is distributed in the dark, especially during the rearing period and just after moving to the laying house.
- Spin feeders during rearing help to reduce feather pecking.
- Because pelleted feed increases the risk of feather pecking unless using spin feeders, a coarse mash is preferred (with added benefits for intestinal health).
- Feeders and drinkers are correctly distributed in the house and feeders are available in the slatted area of the laying house.
- At the onset of production, feed quantity is increased sufficiently quickly to match the increase in egg output.
- Birds have sufficient access to water and have water in their crops 1 h before the lights are turned off.

In addition, house environmental factors are important to improve feather cover.

- Stocking densities higher than recommended will have a detrimental effect on feather quality and increase the risk of feather pecking.

*otto.van.tuijl@planet.nl

- By 21 days of age the birds should have access to the whole rearing area of the house.
- Stimulate feather development by reducing house temperature to 20°C by 28 days of age.
- Ensure good litter quality for dust bathing to maintain feather condition through proper ventilation.
- Fluorescent lights at >100 lux will increase the risk of feather pecking, while incandescent lights reduce the risk.

Other key management factors to reduce abnormal feather loss are as follows.

- Do not place too many males in laying house. By 25 weeks there should be no more than 9% males.
- Ensure that the males and females are at the same level of sexual maturity when they are put together in the laying house to prevent the males damaging the feathers of the females.
- Coccidiosis or necrotic enteritis must be prevented and, if occurring, treated immediately.
- Ensure that birds are handled in a calm way during activities such as weighing and vaccination.
- Prevent mite and/or worm infections and, if found, treat promptly.

INTRODUCTION

All birds, including poultry species, lose and replace their feathers during their lifetime: this is called moulting. Broiler breeders typically moult their feathers twice during rearing and once during production, but different feather tracts and individual feathers moult at different times (Lucas and Stettenheim, 1972). This chapter will discuss factors that trigger abnormal feather loss in broiler breeders, i.e. those losses not caused by the normal moulting process. The chapter will focus on environmental and management factors that affect feathering, as other authors in this volume cover nutritional factors (Chapter 11) and feather pecking (Chapter 3).

As for most birds, feathers are important for broiler breeders as a protection barrier for the skin, thermal insulation and the recognition of flock mates and attraction towards the opposite sex. Feathers become damaged during rearing and production due to mechanical abrasion, feather pecking and mating activity. As a part of general flock management, the feather quality of broiler breeders should be checked regularly. Systems for scoring feather cover are available (Aviagen, 2014).

FIELD OBSERVATIONS

About 20 years ago, reports of poor feathering in broiler breeders started to appear in Europe, including the Netherlands, reaching a peak in 2005. At the time, broiler breeders were still beak trimmed (non-beak-trimmed broiler breeders only became widespread after 2013). An investigation in the Netherlands into the reduction of feather quality seen at this time found several factors and changes that occurred in the same time period that appeared to be associated with the reduction in feather quality. These field observations provided clues as to the management factors that were important in determining good feather quality.

One factor was the breed of broiler: the onset of the problem coincided with a new broiler breed being used in the Netherlands. There was a much higher incidence of feathering problems in the new breed than the standard breed (Table 13.1), though it should be noted that the standard breed did also have some flocks with poor feathers.

At the same time there had been a change from traditional hand-collection nest boxes, using nesting materials such as straw, wood shavings, buckweed or oat hulls, to automated roll-away nest boxes with artificial mats instead of bedding material. There was a higher incidence of feathering problems in the automatic system, but this difference was not statistically significant (Table 13.2).

During the problem period, there was a clear difference between farms supplied by different feed mills. Farms supplied by one feed mill did not show any problems whereas farms supplied by other mills showed either minor (three mills) or severe feathering problems (two mills). The period also coincided with advice given to reduce crude protein levels in breeder diets to improve persistency of production. While the exact nutritional issue was not identified (at least by the author), the feed mills adjusted their specifications and over time the difference between mills disappeared.

There was an increased risk for flocks that had a feathering problem during rearing to have a feathering problem during production (Table 13.3).

It was also during the same period that producers stopped using antibiotic growth promoters and switched from controlling coccidiosis using chemical coccidiostats to coccidiosis vaccination, particularly during the rearing period. As a

Table 13.1. Effect of breed on incidence of feathering problems in Dutch broiler breeder flocks.

	Standard Breed	New Breed
Total flocks	102	49
Problem flocks (%)	9.8	40.8

Chi-squared test $p<0.0001$

Table 13.2. Effect of nest type on incidence of feathering problems in Dutch broiler breeder flocks.

	Traditional	Automatic
Total flocks	28	136
Problem flocks (%)	14.3	22.1

Chi-squared test not significant

Table 13.3. Number of Dutch broiler breeder flocks with problems during rear also having problems during lay.

		Laying	
		No Problem	Problem
Rearing	No problem	24	5
	Problem	5	5

Chi-squared test $p<0.05$

consequence there was an increase in intestinal disorders, resulting in wetter litter and poor feather cover.

The above investigation into the field issues shows that the problem of poor feather cover can be related to many different factors. The rest of this chapter discusses in more detail management factors that affect feather loss, primarily based on field experience. Most of the comments below are based on advice given by primary breeders (Aviagen, 2014, 2016a, b).

RISK FACTORS FOR ABNORMAL FEATHERING

Risk factors can be divided according to the different stages in the life of broiler breeders.

Incubation period

Very little research has been done on the effects of the incubation environment on subsequent feather condition. One study has shown that high incubation temperature will retard feather development both during incubation and during the rearing period (Merat and Cocquerelle, 1991).

Rearing period

Following good management practice as recommended by the primary breeders (e.g. Aviagen, 2018) is essential for good feather development. Particular attention should be paid to:

- correct brooding conditions;
- excessive stocking density, which can lead to feather sucking, feather pulling and eventually aggressive feather pecking;
- ensuring that birds are not confined to the brooding areas for too long and have access to the whole house by 21 days of age; and
- ensuring that house temperatures are reduced following the recommended programme after brooding, targeting 20°C by 28 days of age. Higher temperatures will delay feather development (Lai *et al.*, 2010).

Of key importance is the management of feeders and drinkers. Birds should have access to feed and water immediately after the lights come on in the morning. Broiler breeders are on a controlled feeding regime, which means that all the birds need to be able to feed at the same time. It is essential that recommended feeding space is provided so that all birds can access the feed and obtain the required nutrient intake and to prevent feather damage during feeding. Make sure that there is sufficient space around the feeders so that the birds can access the feed space. Reducing the feeder space by 10% has been found to have a detrimental effect on feather development and quality (Van Emous and Veldkamp, 2009).

Just as important as feeder space is proper feed distribution to ensure that all the feed space contains feed when the birds are feeding. Feed needs to be distributed to all the feeders within 3 min and the feeder hoppers filling the distribution system need to be positioned to achieve this, especially in houses longer than 80 m. If spin feeders are used, feed should be distributed when the lights are off as this will lead to a reduction in gentle feather pecking. As part of the management routine, the birds should regularly be watched feeding to make sure that they all have access to the feed and, if not, action should be taken to remedy the situation.

It is recommended that water is available continuously and controlling water access is not advised. If water access is controlled, it should never be done before 6 weeks of age and the birds' crops should be checked at regular intervals during the day to ensure that they contain some water up to 1 h before lights are off.

Dust bathing is an essential component of feather maintenance and this requires good, dry and friable litter (Pickett, 2008). Maintaining good litter quality at all times is therefore important and immediate action should be taken if the litter becomes caked or wet. In addition to causing feathering problems, wet litter will cause skin problems. Poor litter quality is normally caused by incorrect ventilation, water leaking from drinkers or gut health problems. Proper ventilation is also required to keep ammonia, carbon dioxide and dust levels in the air below recommended levels.

When penning up birds for weighing, grading or vaccination, care must be taken that they do not start to climb on top of each other, as this potentially causes immediate feather damage and any stress could have a long-term effect on feather quality (Zeinstra *et al.*, 2015). The results of stressful events can often be seen in the wing feathers as sections of feather that are not properly formed. Other potential stressors are subclinical coccidiosis or necrotic enteritis, which should be treated promptly. In the case of subclinical coccidiosis, the vaccination procedures should be reviewed and corrected as necessary. In situations of poor intestinal health, providing insoluble grit in the litter at 5, 10 and 15 weeks of age can help.

Good biosecurity on the farm is important to prevent infections such as parvovirus, reovirus and reticuloendotheliosis virus, as these can affect feather development (see also Chapter 7). Vaccination programmes should be designed to meet local disease challenges. Parasites such as red mite or intestinal worms can have an adverse effect on feather quality and if found should be treated immediately and the house thoroughly cleaned and treated before the next flock is placed in the farm (FeatherWel, 2013).

All the factors noted above are important to improve feather quality, but they all require good stockmanship on the farm to identify the issues. Critical signs to watch for during the rearing period are as follows.

- Absence of feathers in the litter from 8 to 10 weeks of age. This is an indicator that feathers are being eaten by the other birds as a source of protein. If this is seen, the nutrition should be reviewed.
- Abnormal screeching noise from the birds. This can be the first sign that feathers are being pulled from birds.
- Birds pecking or chasing each other and poor cover on the flanks. If pecking is before 12 weeks of age, light intensity can be reduced. The use of red instead of white light can also help, as can adding 1 g of salt to 1 l of drinking water for 5 days (Van Niekerk *et al.*, 2013).

Laying period

As in the rearing period, the primary breeder's recommendations for managing the birds should be followed. Many of the recommendations for the rearing period given above should also be followed during the laying period, paying particular attention to:

- feeder space and feed distribution;
- drinker space and water management;
- stocking density;
- litter quality; and
- farm biosecurity.

It is beneficial to use the same type of feeders, drinkers and lighting system on both the rearing and laying farm, as this will allow the birds to settle quickly after transfer and find food and water quickly (Defra, 2005). For the first 3–4 weeks after transfer it is important to distribute the feed to the feeders when the lights are off. Avoid high light intensities (>60 lux), especially with fluorescent lights, as it increases the risk of feather sucking, aggressive interactions and general nervousness in the flock.

During lay a major cause of feather damage is due to mating activity (Van Emous, 2009). When the males and females are moved into the laying house they must be at the same stage of sexual maturity to prevent the males becoming overly aggressive to the females at the start of production. Similarly, the correct number of males should be placed into the flock of females: if there are too many males the females will be mated too frequently, resulting in excessive feather damage, particularly on the back and thighs. If a female's feather cover is insufficient, it will hide away from the males and fertility of the flock will decline.

Feeding levels during production need to be carefully managed to ensure that adequate energy is provided to maintain egg production, body weight and feather cover. If the bird goes into a negative energy balance, it adversely affects both egg production and feather cover. Special care needs to be taken post peak egg production, when feed levels are normally reduced as egg mass output declines. Poorly feathered flocks will also require a higher level of feed intake, due to the higher heat loss from reduced thermal insulation, typically about 3 g feed/day for every 1 point of feather score (Van Emous and Veldkamp, 2009). Higher feed intakes will increase the protein intake, which can have a negative impact on fertility and hatch and will increase feed cost.

If feathering deteriorates during production, consider: (i) reducing mating ratio; (ii) filling feeder systems in the dark; (iii) using feed distribution time of less than 3 min; (iv) raising the house temperature; (v) adjusting feed allocation; and (vi) checking the water supply.

SUMMARY

Ensuring that all birds have proper access to the correct quantity and quality of feed and sufficient clean drinking water in combination with the right environmental conditions, including good litter quality at all stages of life, are important factors to ensure good feather cover at all times. Observation of the birds under these conditions is an essential part of standard management procedures.

REFERENCES

Aviagen (2014) *A Practical Guide to Managing Feather Cover in Broiler Breeder Females*. Available at: http://eu.aviagen.com/assets/Tech_Center/Ross_Tech_Articles/RossTechNoteFeathering2014-EN.pdf (accessed 12 October 2018).

Aviagen (2016a) *Feathering in Broiler Breeder Females*. Available at: http://eu.aviagen.com/assets/Tech_Center/Broiler_Breeder_Tech_Articles/English/Feathering-in-Broiler-Breeeder-Females-EN-2016.pdf (accessed 12 October 2018).

Aviagen (2016b) *Management of Broiler Breeders in the Absence of Beak Treatment*. Available at: http://eu.aviagen.com/assets/Tech_Center/Broiler_Breeder_Tech_Articles/English/AviagenBrief-BeakTreatment-EN-2016.pdf (accessed 12 October 2018).

Aviagen (2018) *Parent Stock Management Handbook*. Available at: http://eu.aviagen.com/techcenter/download/19/RossPSHandBook2018.pdf (accessed 16 October 2018).

Defra (2005) *A Guide to the Practical Management of Feather Pecking & Cannibalism in Free Range Laying Hens*. ADAS Poultry Group, Department for Environment, Food & Rural Affairs, London. Available at: https://assets.publishing.service.gov.uk/government/uploads/system/uploads/attachment_data/file/69374/pb10596-feather-pecking-050309.pdf (accessed 12 October 2018).

FeatherWel (2013) *Improving Feather Cover. A Guide to Reducing the Risk of Injurious Pecking Occurring in Non-cage Laying Hens*. University of Bristol. Available at: http://www.featherwel.org/Portals/3/Documents/Improving%20feather%20cover%20advice%20guide.pdf (accessed 12 October 2018).

Lai, P.W., Liang, J.B., Hsia, L.C., Loh, T.C. and Ho, Y.W. (2010) Effects of varying dietary zinc levels and environmental temperatures on the growth performance, feathering score and feather mineral concentrations of broiler chicks. *Asian–Australasian Journal of Animal Sciences* 23(7), 937–945.

Lucas, A.M. and Stettenheim, P.R. (1972) *Avian Anatomy: Integument*. Agriculture Handbook 362. Department of Agriculture. US Government Printing Office, Washington, DC.

Merat, P. and Cocquerelle, G. (1991) Effects of slightly higher or lower than normal incubation temperatures on embryonic mortality, posthatching performances and feathering. *Annales de Zootechnie* 40, 67–72.

Pickett, H. (2008) *Controlled Feather Pecking & Cannibalism in Laying Hens Without Beak Trimming*. A Compassion in World Farming report. Available at: https://www.ciwf.org.uk/includes/documents/cm_docs/2009/c/controlling_feather_pecking_and_cannibalism_without_beak_trimming.pdf (accessed 12 October 2018).

Van Emous, R.A. (2009) Strak in het verenpak. *Pluimveehouderij* 39, 30–31.

Van Emous, R.A. and Veldkamp, T. (2009) Hongerige veren. *Pluimveehouderij* 39, 36–37.

Van Niekerk, T.G.C.M., de Jong, I.C., van Krimpen, M.M., Reuvekamp, B.F.J., van Tuijl, O. and Bestman, M. (2013) *Noodmaatregelen tegen pikkerij*. Livestock Research Wageningen UR – 32, Lelystad, the Netherlands. Available at: http://edepot.wur.nl/283863 (accessed 12 October 2018).

Zeinstra, E.C., Oeben, L., van der Staay, F.J., and Nordquist, R.E. (2015) Methoden voor de bepaling van corticosteron in veren. *Biotechniek* 54, 17–22.

CHAPTER 14
Business Opportunities with the Integument

Stephen Lister*

Crowshall Veterinary Services LLP, Attleborough, Norfolk, UK

ABSTRACT

The integument is an important organ system protecting the bird by acting as a barrier between the external environment and internal body systems, providing thermal insulation and for regulation of water loss. Arguably, as a result, the major business opportunity with the integument is to maintain the integrity of feathers, skin, scales and foot pads to protect and enhance bird health and performance, and through this boost economic return at processing. Feather cover and foot pad integrity are also used as proxy measures of animal husbandry, management, environmental control and bird health and are increasingly important as welfare outcome measures. In this way the integument acts as an important indicator of bird health and welfare. At processing, the harvesting of avian feathers, down, feet, skin and tongues can offer further business opportunities for by-products that would otherwise be considered as waste. The most profitable and widespread use of the integument as a by-product is the use of feather and down for bedding and clothing. Historically feathers were seen as an essential fashion accessory, often commanding prices of more than their weight in gold. Less obvious uses have been as an animal protein source, pet food, fertilizer, bacterial culture medium, enzyme production and adhesives. Recent interest has been in the production of biodegradable composite plastics from processed feathers. Chicken feet (paws) and duck feet, together with duck tongues, combs and wattles, have the potential to satisfy an increasing export opportunity for markets where these food choices are popular. This chapter will discuss some of these opportunities and factors that could adversely affect quality.

*salister@crowshall.co.uk

INTRODUCTION

The integument is an important organ system in all avian species. It includes the feathers, skin and scale of shanks and feet. Primarily it is the defence barrier between the external environment and internal body systems of the bird. It provides thermal insulation and allows regulation of water loss. An intact, unblemished skin is essential to the visual appearance of many fresh or frozen poultry products. In addition, this visual appearance can be used as a welfare outcome indicator for veterinarians, processors, quality control assessment and by the end consumer in their purchasing decisions of whole birds, portions and other further processed products.

There is also a commercial business imperative for high-quality feathers, skin, feet and tongues.

Disease prevention and protection

As well as being important to the processor, maintenance of the integrity of feathers, skin, scales and foot pads serves to protect and enhance bird health and performance. The defence barrier can aid in preventing an assortment of disease and pathological challenges and damage. These include: (i) viral, bacterial, parasitic, fungal, mycotoxins; (ii) nutritional; (iii) physical/trauma; (iv) neoplasia; and (v) genetic.

Defence barrier between external environment and internal body systems

An intact integument provides a physical barrier, with the presence of skin surface lysozymes. The skin and feathers are important for thermal insulation and in the regulation of water loss.

A welfare outcome indicator

Feather cover and foot pad integrity are used as proxy measures of animal husbandry, stockmanship, management, environmental control, bird health and welfare. A range of factors may be used to assess bird quality both on farm and at processing. These factors include: (i) feather cover; (ii) pododermatitis; (iii) hock burn; (iv) breast blisters (jelly belly, button ulcers); and (v) skin tears.

POTENTIAL BUSINESS OPPORTUNITIES FOR BY-PRODUCTS

Harvesting of avian feathers, down, feet, skin and tongues, which might otherwise be considered as unwelcome by-products of processing carcasses for production of edible whole carcasses, portions and further processed products, can give economic return on such products themselves as well as reducing rendering or other disposal costs.

In more recent years, the most lucrative by-products have been feather and down for bedding and clothing, though historically feathers were a sought-after fashion accessory. There has also been a domestic or export market for high-quality chicken feet (or paws), duck feet, tongues, combs and wattles. Other outlets have included their use as an alternative animal protein source. Feather meal and hydrolysed proteins can be used as an alternative animal protein source for livestock diets or pet food. There is some interest in these animal proteins as fertilizer, bacterial culture media, enzyme production, adhesives and most recently as sustainable biodegradable plastics.

The use of the integument in these circumstances can depend on economic, cultural or phyto-sanitary considerations. This can often result in such materials being considered a costly waste product, though any outlets, even for products of minimal value, are preferable to the costs of disposal and may also enhance the sustainability credentials of the industry.

SKIN

The skin is considered an integral part of whole carcass appearance. An 'A' grade carcass is one free of blemishes, skin tears, breast blisters or ulcers and hock burn. Cellulitis conditions, variously described as cherry hip, skin necrosis and infectious process, can affect skin and the underlying muscle meat. Skin-on products are popular, especially as fresh options at retail outlets, and mean that whole birds or portions are 'poultry on show' and consumers will instinctively choose clean, unblemished products. All such blemishes reduce value and this applies equally to chicken, turkey, duck, goose and game birds.

High-quality skin also has an importance in further processing as a natural adhesive and former of further processed products

FEATHERS

For many years ostrich, duck, goose and chicken feathers have been harvested for commercial gain. They have been used in duvets, pillows and increasingly for high-quality, lightweight insulated jackets. Mature duck breeder feather tends to be more highly sought after than commercial meat feather, due to its enhanced insulating properties.

Historically feathers were also used for fletching arrows, as fishing lures and for the production of quill pens. Indeed, the word 'pen' is thought to be derived from *penna*, the Latin for feather.

Although now used far less as a fashion accessory, in 1903 hunters were paid US$32 per ounce of ostrich plumes, making them worth about twice their weight in gold. As a result, feathers used to be worth, weight for weight, the same as diamonds.

To serve this demand, domestication of ostrich rearing for feathers has been significant in South Africa since the 1830s. This increased from the 1940s, due to commercialization for skin and ostrich leather production. South Africa still remains the main producer in the world, currently slaughtering up to 250,000 birds each year for meat, leather and feathers. Globally over 400,000 birds are reared in up to 100 different countries, but notably in Central and South America.

Breeding and rearing ostrich is not easy, requiring high standards of stockmanship, suitable climate and adequate space for birds that prosper in isolated groups. Ostrich meat, which was once considered a by-product of feather harvesting, has become a popular product in its own right. The meat produced from ostrich is described as 'fat free' and is low in cholesterol and saturated fatty acids. Mature birds are slaughtered at about 12 months of age with a liveweight of about 100 kg. Some 15 square feet (1.4 m^2) of leather can be harvested from a large male, with increased value after processing and tanning.

Feathers in Europe

Europe may produce some 1,200,000 t of feather, down and feather meal each year from a variety of avian species. The price is very volatile over time and is very sensitive to supply and demand, making it difficult to assess its true monetary value. A major issue for livestock production is that feathers tend to have a low nutritive value as a protein source. There are also issues in some countries of the legalities as an animal protein by-product for feeding back to other livestock. These difficulties have led to interest in other commercial opportunities, which have included: (i) bio-composites (combining with polypropylene to produce plastic bioresin with lower carbon footprint); (ii) feather-based bacterial culture media; (iii) enyzme production; and (iv) adhesives.

Welfare considerations of plucking, harvesting and gathering

For many years it has been considered that the live plucking of ducks or geese is an unacceptable procedure. The live plucking of geese was specifically considered by the European Food Safety Authority in 2010 (EFSA, 2010).

EFSA identified that up to 99% of feather harvesting is as a by-product of food processing, so only 1% is gathered from live geese. The gathering (harvesting or collecting) of goose feathers has been done for 2000 years. Gathering is defined as removing feathers that are ripe due to moulting, referring to brushing or combing action to remove feathers/down ready to fall out, specifically without causing bleeding or tissue damage. Plucking, on the other hand, refers to the targeted pulling of feathers. EFSA concluded that plucking was an unacceptable activity as the damage represents the ability to cause 'unnecessary pain, suffering or disease'. This may be manifested as bloody feather quills, skin injuries or posture changes from plucking or mortality, or more severely, dislocated or broken bones due to rough catching and handling.

Feather harvesting

Feathers harvested at poultry slaughter and processing, predominantly for pillows, duvets or feather meal, can attract a price of up to £30/t, depending on its quality and source.

It is possible to harvest up to 100 g of washed and dried feather per standard duck carcass, and up to 250 g from geese. This equates to approximately 5% of adult body weight. Value is difficult to assess, due to volatile market conditions, especially associated with export considerations and aspects of supply and demand from different markets. Some current estimates in the UK are between £1.50 to £2.00/kg of washed, clean duck feather. Goose feather can attract a price of four to five times that. Most product is exported to the Far East and increasingly the USA, with some smaller European customers. It is expensive to transport feather in volume and so usually this is done as compressed bales in full shipping containers

Feather meal

There is currently no market for feather meal in UK animal feeds, due to issues over processed animal protein being banned for feeding to other livestock species since the emergence of bovine spongiform encephalopathy (BSE). There is a pet-food market, though feet are probably the preferred protein source. Outside the EU, feather meal is more regularly used in animal feeds, with up to 5% feed inclusion. Feather meal is high in protein (80%) but most of this is as keratin. As a result, aggressive processing is required to hydrolyse the protein content, usually via a pressure-cooking process with live steam. Even then the hydrolysed meal has a poor amino acid profile, especially for methionine, lysine and histidine. Therefore supply and processing costs must be economic to compete with other protein sources such as soybean meal. Another potential market for feather meal has been for mink production in Russia and Scandinavia.

FEET AND TONGUES

There is potentially a major export market for duck and chicken feet and tongues to the Far East. There are significant quality requirements and avian diseases, predominantly fears in relation to avian influenza, are a major barrier to trade. As with feathers, ongoing issues of supply and demand strongly affect price and sales. Quality is considered important and feet with pododermatitis, blisters or dirty condition are downgraded to animal by-products (ABP), as they are not fit for human consumption. In the UK the feet must be washed to remove visible contamination and are then graded as A (blemish free), B (slight marking) or C (extensive marking or calluses).

Quality may be improved by heated water treatment to remove the surface epithelium. Product can then be sold fresh or frozen, locally or for export, with prices ranging from £0.45 to £0.90/kg.

Feet are very important for cuisines in China, Indonesia, Korea, Thailand, Malaysia and increasingly other countries. They may be prepared fried, steamed, stewed or marinated. In China, high-quality feet can be worth, weight for weight, the same as frozen chicken breast. In 2000, Hong Kong traded 420,000 t with an estimated value of US$230 million. Some estimates suggest that the UK market for export could be £30 million if conditions are right and trade issues can be addressed.

CONCLUSIONS

There are a number of important business opportunities with the integument. This will continue to include feathers, skin, feet, wattles and combs, either individually or as part of the quality of whole carcasses, portions and further processed products. There are already established markets for feet and feathers from ducks, geese and chickens. Quality, availability and logistics remain vital to servicing this market, which is very dependent on global supply-and-demand pressures. Unfortunately, the disease status of different countries is a major barrier to free trade. This is especially relevant with respect to the current global issues being experienced in many countries with avian influenza. This is likely to have the major influence on trade for some time to come and is likely to focus attention on more local and secure sources of products.

REFERENCE

EFSA (2010) Scientific opinion on the practice of harvesting (collecting) feathers from live geese for down production. *EFSA Journal* 8(11), 1886. doi: 10.2903/j.efsa.2010.1886

INDEX

Note: Page numbers in **bold** type refer to **figures**
Page numbers in *italic* type refer to *tables*